ALSO BY DR. JOSEPH MERCOLA

*Fat for Fuel**

Effortless Healing

The No-Grain Diet

Take Control of Your Health

Sweet Deception

Dark Deception

The Great Bird Flu Hoax

Generation XL

Healthy Recipes for Your Nutritional Type

———

ALSO BY PETE EVANS

The Complete Gut Health Cookbook

The Paleo Chef

*Available from Hay House
Please visit:

Hay House USA: www.hayhouse.com®
Hay House Australia: www.hayhouse.com.au
Hay House UK: www.hayhouse.co.uk
Hay House South Africa: www.hayhouse.co.za
Hay House India: www.hayhouse.co.in

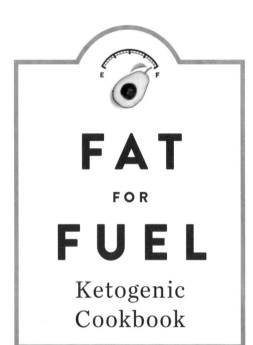

FAT

FOR

FUEL

Ketogenic
Cookbook

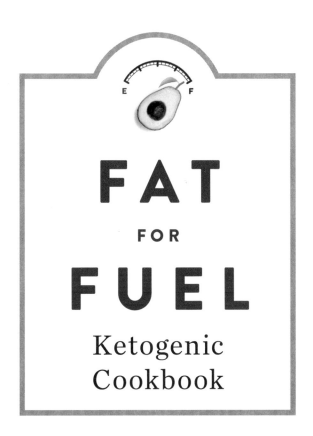

FAT FOR FUEL

Ketogenic Cookbook

Recipes and Ketogenic Keys to Health
from a World-Class Doctor and
an Internationally Renowned Chef

DR. JOSEPH MERCOLA
& PETE EVANS

HAY HOUSE, INC.
Carlsbad, California • New York City
London • Sydney • Johannesburg
Vancouver • New Delhi

FOUNTAINDALE PUBLIC LIBRARY

300 West Briarcliff Road
Bolingbrook, IL 60440-2894
(630) 759-2102

Copyright © 2017 by Joseph Mercola and Pete Evans

Published and distributed in the United States by: Hay House, Inc.: www.hayhouse.com® • **Published and distributed in Australia by:** Hay House Australia Pty. Ltd.: www.hayhouse.com.au • **Published and distributed in the United Kingdom by:** Hay House UK, Ltd.: www.hayhouse.co.uk • **Published and distributed in the Republic of South Africa by:** Hay House SA (Pty), Ltd.: www.hayhouse.co.za • **Distributed in Canada by:** Raincoast Books: www.raincoast.com • **Published in India by:** Hay House Publishers India: www.hayhouse.co.in

Cover design: Laura Palese
Interior design: Riann Bender
Interior photos: William Meppem, Steve Brown, Rob Palmer, and Mark Roper
Food Stylists: Lucy Tweed and Deborah Kaloper
Indexer: Jay Kreider
Images used under license from Shutterstock.com: Pages viii, x, 17, 26, 28, 32, 34, and 68

All rights reserved. No part of this book may be reproduced by any mechanical, photographic, or electronic process, or in the form of a phonographic recording; nor may it be stored in a retrieval system, transmitted, or otherwise be copied for public or private use—other than for "fair use" as brief quotations embodied in articles and reviews—without prior written permission of the publisher.

The authors of this book do not dispense medical advice or prescribe the use of any technique as a form of treatment for physical, emotional, or medical problems without the advice of a physician, either directly or indirectly. The intent of the authors is only to offer information of a general nature to help you in your quest for emotional, physical, and spiritual well-being. In the event you use any of the information in this book for yourself, the authors and the publisher assume no responsibility for your actions.

Cataloging-in-Publication Data is on file at the Library of Congress

Hardcover ISBN: 978-1-4019-5541-0

10 9 8 7 6 5 4 3 2 1
1st edition, November 2017

Printed in the United States of America

SUSTAINABLE FORESTRY INITIATIVE
Certified Chain of Custody
Promoting Sustainable Forestry
www.sfiprogram.org
SFI-01268

SFI label applies to the text stock

I dedicate this book to my mom.
Her sudden passing right before its publication
has forever changed me.
I love you, Mom.

— Dr. Mercola

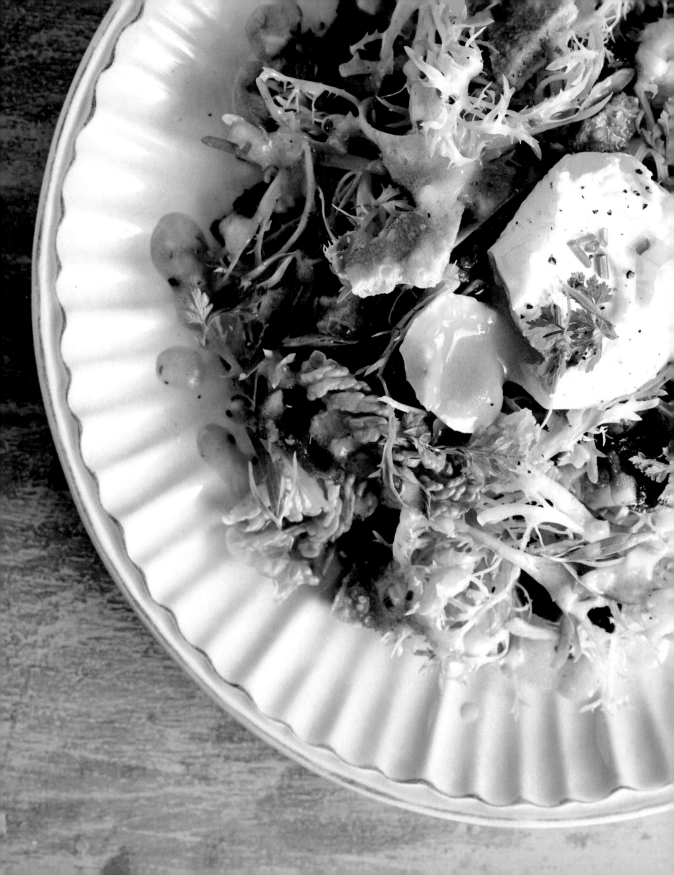

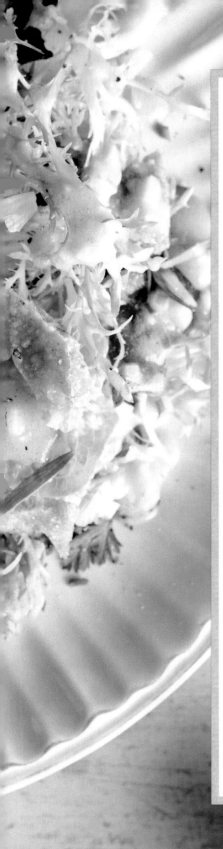

CONTENTS

· ·

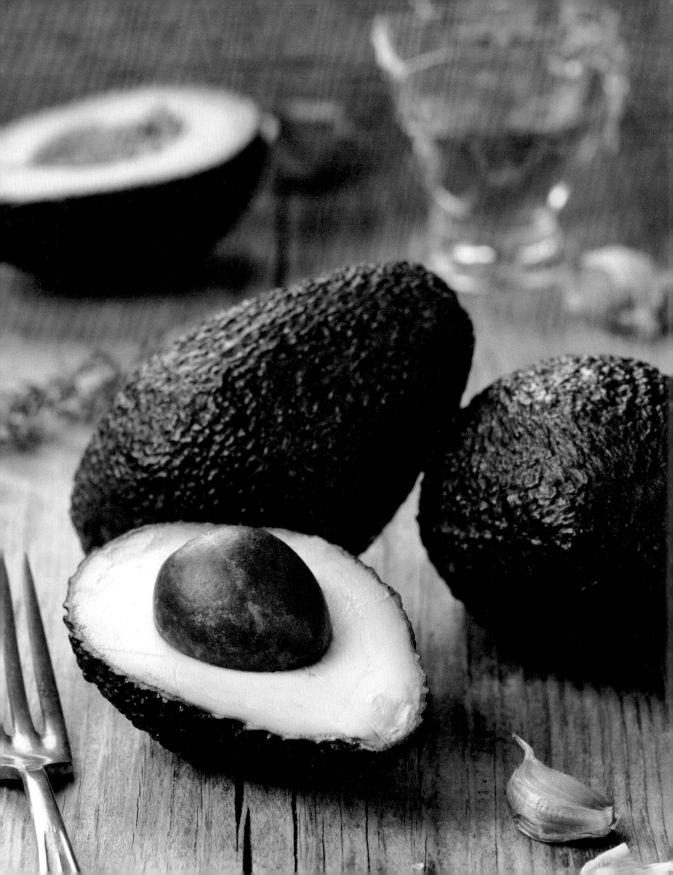

AUTHOR'S NOTE

I believe that *Fat for Fuel* is the most important book I have ever written, because making the shift away from relying on glucose as your primary source of energy to burning fat has such profound benefits for your health—from shedding excess weight to helping ward off and fight the chronic diseases that are afflicting us in ever greater numbers, including diabetes and cancer. That's why I was so happy to see the book become the number-one-selling nonfiction book in May 2017 according to *The Wall Street Journal* and *USA Today*. By achieving this ranking it means that many people now have the nutritional knowledge they need to take control of their health.

But with as much information as I packed into *Fat for Fuel*, it still didn't provide the total picture. That book told you *what* changes to make to your diet and provided the details that explain *why* to do it. You still need to know *how* to implement the dietary changes and strategies. This cookbook shows you how.

The recipes included on these pages will give you the inspiration as well as the step-by-step instructions you need to start experiencing not only how good it feels to eat a fat-burning diet, but also how incredibly delicious it can be. Where *Fat for Fuel* speaks to your head, *Fat for Fuel Ketogenic Cookbook* appeals directly to your taste buds and your stomach.

To make the recipes as appealing as possible—so that you would be compelled by your senses to adopt to the diet as well as by your head—I reached out to the Australian celebrity chef Pete Evans. A restaurateur, household chef, and author in his own right, Pete shares a dedication to eating healthy, fat-burning foods that are as scrumptious as they are nutritious. Together, we can deliver the full package of research-backed medical advice and kitchen-tested recipes that will help empower you to make the shift to fat-burning and reap the powerful health benefits such a metabolic transition can bring.

It is my sincere hope that this book becomes dog-eared and food-splattered as you use it to cook your way to radiant health.

Dr. Joseph Mercola

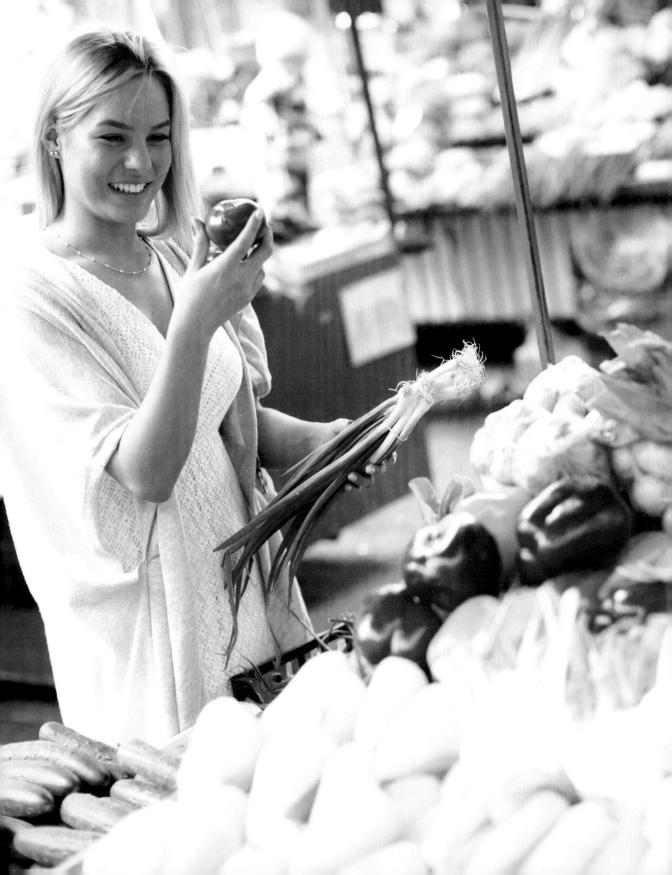

INTRODUCTION

The age-old question "What's for dinner?" is one of the most important questions you can ask yourself. Why? Because when Hippocrates wrote, "Let food be thy medicine and medicine be thy food," he was sharing an elemental truth: if your food isn't contributing to your health, it's contributing to your illness.

Despite the overwhelming evidence of food's healing powers, you aren't likely to get much nutritional guidance from your doctor, if you get any at all. This isn't necessarily your doctor's fault—most medical schools fail to provide students any formal training on proper nutrition and how it can prevent a wide range of diseases in the first place.[1] Most medical students are schooled in treating symptoms (with a pharmaceutical drug) rather than treating the disease. You may receive guidance to lose a little weight by watching your calories, but that's as far as the typical nutritional guidance goes.

I was once one of these doctors. Despite an early interest in nutrition—my fellow medical students nicknamed me "Dr. Fiber" in the late 1970s for my devotion to eating fiber-rich foods—my thinking had been very much indoctrinated by the "fix it with a prescription" model of mainstream medicine.

WHEN FOOD ISN'T MEDICINE

Because I am a passionate lifelong learner, I'm absolutely committed to staying on top of current health research. I regularly attend and teach at postgraduate seminars, read an average of two to three books and dozens of studies a week, and interview leading experts on health and nutrition.

My understanding of nutrition continues to evolve. Since my book *Fat for Fuel* came out in May 2017, I have refined my thinking. This is thanks to the work of Dr. Steven Gundry, author of the book *The Plant Paradox*. Dr. Gundry has studied the negative effects of lectins—proteins that occur naturally in an estimated 30 percent of fresh foods. They serve to protect the plant while it's growing, but once eaten, they can wreak havoc inside your body. These proteins are a wondrous self-defense mechanism for the plant; they can selectively bind to specific types of harmful molecules, such as fungi, and render them powerless, protecting the plant from attack. Inside your body, however, lectins can bind to any number of carbohydrates. The lectins found in wheat, for example, bind to specific receptor sites on your intestinal mucosal cells and interfere with the absorption of nutrients across your intestinal wall. In other words, they can act like an "antinutrient," exerting a detrimental effect on your gut microbiome and promoting inflammation. This is definitely not food as medicine!

There are numerous types of lectins, and not all of them are harmful—we are still developing our understanding of them, and controversy and confusion surround them. Still, this is one example of how we all need to be careful to not ever think that we know all there is to know about nutrition and food. There is so much to be uncovered and understood.

TASTE MATTERS TOO

As vital a role as food plays in health, it is more than just a nutrient delivery system. Food enhances your enjoyment of life and gives you an opportunity to commune with people you know and love. Beyond that, cooking food is a creative outlet and an act of love for whoever will eat it—whether that's you or other people.

That's why I am so excited and honored to work with Pete Evans, an internationally renowned chef, restaurateur, and cookbook author, on this cookbook. Our goal is to deliver a synergistic balance of crucial nutritional insight *and* delectable recipes. It's our intention to bring you the best of all possible worlds

in this book—some nutrition books are too technical, and some cookbooks rely too heavily on pretty photographs without offering any educational substance. We aim to empower you with the information you need to select the right foods for you, to inspire you by showing you how delicious and nourishing these foods can be, and to tell you exactly how to create them for yourself.

On the pages that follow, you'll get the distilled version of why diet matters so much to health. You'll learn not only what to eat, but also how to improve your digestion, ward off or radically reduce type 2 diabetes, choose better beverages, and support your diet with a few well-chosen supplements so that you can find and maintain the weight that's right for you as you also optimize your overall health. I'll also share some surprising insights on cooking methods that will help you make the food you prepare as health-supportive as it can possibly be. Then Pete will come in and share his best recipes for foods that support fat burning. You never knew how delicious supporting your health can be!

I want to congratulate you for seeking to upgrade your understanding of nutrition by reading this book—none of us will ever be done learning about the best ways to feed and nourish our bodies. I hope this book will lead to many memorable and delicious meals around your table as well as radiant health over the long term.

PART I

KETOGENIC KEYS TO HEALTH

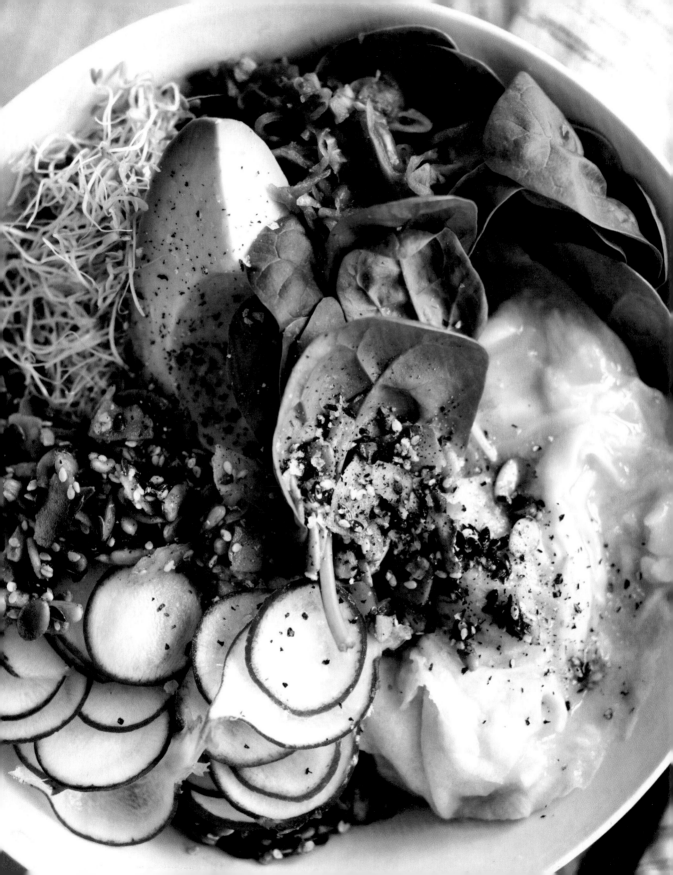

UNCOVER THE ROOT CAUSE OF DISEASE

In my decades as a family physician and in the 20 years since I launched my website, Mercola.com, my ultimate aim has always been the same: to empower you to realize that it is completely within your control to correct the root causes of obesity and disease. You don't need a prescription or expensive treatments. What you *do* need is to change what and when you eat. I know this may not seem like an easy fix, and I can't promise that it doesn't require some mental and physical effort. But when you consider that it is something you can start today and that it doesn't require anyone else's permission to implement, I think you'll agree that the empowerment strategy outlined in these pages more than makes up for any effort required on your part. Just by picking up and reading this book, you're already well on your way.

Addressing the underlying causes of illness isn't as big or complicated a task as it might seem, as the most common diseases—including obesity, diabetes, heart disease, Alzheimer's, and cancer—all share a common root. They are all triggered and exacerbated by insulin and leptin resistance that results in mitochondrial dysfunction. And insulin and leptin resistance are a direct result of your diet.

Insulin is a hormone released by your pancreas to keep your blood sugar at the appropriate level. Your body has approximately one gallon of blood in it, and of that gallon, only

one teaspoon should be sugar—if that. Even a minor rise in blood sugar above this level is dangerous. In fact, if your blood sugar level were to rise to one tablespoon, you would likely go into a hypoglycemic coma and die if not treated.

If you consume a diet consistently high in sugar and grains (net carbohydrates), your blood glucose levels will be correspondingly high. Over time your body will become desensitized to insulin and require more and more of it to maintain normal blood sugar levels. This desensitization is called insulin resistance.

Leptin, on the other hand, is a hormone that helps you regulate your appetite. It's produced by your fat cells and sends the signal to your brain that you've eaten enough. The more fat you have stored in your cells, the more leptin you produce. The problem is that, over time, your brain can become desensitized to leptin's signals, known as leptin resistance. As you become increasingly resistant to the effects of leptin, you end up eating more than you need to stay healthy.

Insulin and leptin resistance trigger biochemical cascades that not only make your body hold on to fat, but increase inflammation and cellular damage. This may seem like bad news, but it is actually very exciting because it means that whether you're struggling with excess weight or with chronic health issues—or both—there's likely one simple protocol that will easily address these issues. You won't need a different set of strategies to address each condition, which significantly simplifies the road to improving your health.

CYCLICAL NUTRITIONAL KETOSIS CAN REVERSE INSULIN AND LEPTIN RESISTANCE

Insulin and leptin resistance develop as a result of consuming too many net carbohydrates (total carbs minus fiber) and/or too much protein. Since processed foods, grains, and meat are the staples of the American diet *and* the primary sources of increased insulin and leptin, eating less of these foods is crucial to healing your insulin and leptin resistance. It leads to losing weight and radically improving your health.

By eating a healthy high-fat, low-carbohydrate, and adequate-protein diet, you eventually enter into a condition called nutritional ketosis, in which your body burns fat as its primary fuel rather than glucose. More and more studies are confirming the concept that nutritional ketosis can be a fundamental, effective strategy to address a long list of health problems.

In fact, emerging scientific evidence suggests a high-fat, low-net-carb, and adequate-protein diet (in other words, a diet that keeps you in cyclical nutritional ketosis) is ideal for most people. This is the diet that I outline in great detail in my book *Fat for Fuel*, and it's what I recommend for most people who would like to optimize their health.

It's important to note that I'm not advocating long-term, uninterrupted nutritional ketosis, which can actually be counterproductive: if insulin levels get *too* low, it can paradoxically drive up your blood sugar. Why does this happen? Insulin's main function is to suppress the manufacture of glucose by the liver (hepatic gluconeogenesis). So if your insulin levels remain low for a long period of time, your liver won't get the message to stop making glucose, and this will drive up your blood sugar levels. The way to avoid this situation is to cycle in and out of nutritional ketosis, fasting one day a week and feasting one or two days a week, eating double or triple your typical amount of net carbs. This approach helps you regain your metabolic flexibility, meaning your ability to burn glucose and to burn fat. Most people have lost the ability to burn fat altogether. Attaining and maintaining nutritional ketosis for several months will help reignite your ability to burn fat for fuel. From there, you will move in and out of it for long-term health.

Beyond resolving insulin and leptin resistance, there are a number of other important health benefits of nutritional ketosis. Perhaps the longest-known and most-researched is the ketogenic diet's use as a treatment for seizures, especially in cases that are resistant to drugs.

Even if you don't have a major illness, there are many reasons why you should consider a cyclical ketogenic diet, including:

- **Losing weight**

   Adopting a cyclical ketogenic diet is one of the most effective ways to lose excess body fat because it helps your body burn stored fat for fuel. It's counterintuitive because we've been so indoctrinated into thinking that fat is fattening. But when you reduce your net carb intake and optimize your blood sugar levels, you improve insulin and leptin resistance and the ability of your mitochondria—the small organelles that are essentially your body's energy generator—to burn fuel efficiently.

In one study, obese test subjects were given either a low-carb ketogenic diet or a low-fat diet. After 24 weeks, researchers noted that the low-carb group had lost more weight (9.4 kilograms) than the low-fat group (4.8 kilograms).[1]

- **Lowering inflammation**

  By eliminating sugar from your diet, you're decreasing your risk of developing chronic inflammation throughout your body—a major risk factor for nearly every chronic disease.

  When you stop eating sugar and follow a cyclical ketogenic diet, you train your body to burn fat, which is a "cleaner" fuel than sugar. In other words, your body can burn ketones (a form of fuel manufactured by the liver from stored or dietary fat) far more efficiently and generate far fewer reactive oxygen species (ROS)—unstable molecules that go on to form free radicals—than when it burns glucose for fuel. You've likely heard the term *free radicals* before; it refers to unstable

molecules that damage your mitochondrial and nuclear DNA, protein, and cell membranes. Simply put: sugar creates far more ROS. When eaten in excess, it causes premature degeneration from excessive oxidative stress.

- **Reducing risk of cancer and treating existing cancer**

  All of your cells, including cancer cells, can use glucose as fuel. However, unlike your healthy cells, cancer cells do not have the metabolic flexibility to adapt to using fat as an energy source. Once your body enters a state of nutritional ketosis, precancerous and cancer cells become impaired and far more susceptible to being eliminated by apoptosis, the process your body uses to eliminate disease and damaged cells.

- **Increasing muscle mass**

  When you stop eating high levels of net carbs, your body transitions to burning fat and producing water-soluble fats known as ketones, which are then used by your cells for energy. When optimized in cyclical ketosis, ketones help promote muscle mass, which is good whether you're an athlete, an elderly person, or someone who is simply seeking to be more fit and strong.

- **Normalizing appetite**

  Persistent hunger can cause you to consume more calories than you can burn, which can eventually lead to weight gain. A cyclical ketogenic diet can help you avoid this problem because reducing net carbohydrate consumption can reduce hunger symptoms. In one study, participants who were given a low-carbohydrate diet had reduced appetites, helping them lose weight more easily.[2]

- **Lowering insulin levels**

  By dramatically reducing the number of net carbs you consume, you also lower your blood sugar level, which then leads to lower levels of insulin and leptin. In a study published in *Nutrition & Metabolism*, researchers noted that diabetics who ate low-carbohydrate ketogenic diets were able to significantly reduce their dependency on diabetes medication and in some cases even reverse the disease.[3]

- **Improving mental clarity**

  Your brain works better when operating on a more efficient fuel (i.e., fat or ketones). Many times, improved cognition is one of the first things people notice after starting a ketogenic diet.

- **Taming junk food cravings**

  Although it can take a bit of time and discipline to transition your body to burn fat as your primary fuel, once you've made the switch you simply don't feel deprived. Now that your body has the flexibility to burn fat once your glycogen (sugar) stores run low, you don't need to grab sugar to refuel it.

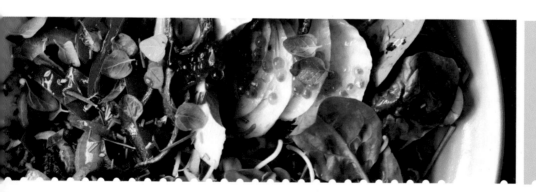

IT'S ALL ABOUT YOUR METABOLISM

A cyclical ketogenic diet provides so many health benefits because it works on a cellular level to repair your metabolism. When I say "metabolism," I don't mean the rate at which you digest your food. I'm talking about the process that happens within your cells in your mitochondria.

The process that converts the reduced form of food you eat and the air you breathe into energy happens in the electron transport chain on the inner membrane of your mitochondria. The energy molecules that are created, which are known as adenosine triphosphate (ATP), allow the efficient transfer of energy to your cells. Without generating ATP you cannot survive at all.

Optimizing your mitochondrial function—and preventing mitochondrial dysfunction by making sure your body is burning fat for fuel—is extremely important for health and disease prevention.

Mitochondria manufacture ATP in a process called oxidative phosphorylation. However, this process also produces by-products that are harmful to your cells, including reactive oxygen species (ROS), which can then generate dangerous free radicals. Free radicals are molecules with unpaired electrons that attack and damage healthy DNA, proteins, and cell membranes, causing a ripple effect that keeps creating more and more free radicals and contributing to aging and disease.

Free radicals also serve as important signaling molecules, so you need to avoid indiscriminately suppressing important baseline levels with excessive antioxidants. Rather, you want to make sure that you aren't producing *excessive* free radicals. And the most effective way to do that is to teach your body to burn fat for fuel and generate far cleaner-burning ketones.

How a Low-Carb, High-Fat, and Adequate-Protein Diet Fosters Health

Eating healthy fat is also beneficial to your mitochondria because it contributes to the building blocks of your cellular membranes. If your cell membranes are impaired, you will invariably have compromised health. So dietary fat serves two purposes: it is a fuel, and it's also a foundational structural component of your biology.

Beyond eating more high-quality fat and fewer net carbs, you also should moderate how much protein you consume. Granted, protein is an essential building block of your body and you need some, but if you consistently eat more than your body requires to run and repair itself, the excess protein will stimulate an ancient metabolic signaling pathway called mTOR (mammalian target of rapamycin), which can orchestrate insulin, leptin, and other crucial hormones. mTOR is responsible for triggering either growth or repair, depending on whether it is stimulated or inhibited. Because cancer is essentially growth gone wild, having an upregulated mTOR pathway can increase your risk of cancer and other degenerative diseases.

So the ideal ratio of macronutrients for a ketogenic diet is high fat, low net carb, and adequate protein. This breakdown of nutrients is very different from the typical American diet and a big reason why I am so excited to partner with Pete Evans to provide you with delicious recipes that are designed to help you achieve the proper balance of macronutrients.

The key to success on a high-fat diet is to eat high-quality, healthy fats, not the fats most commonly found in the American diet, such as hydrogenated fats and refined vegetable oils, which are present in so many processed foods, salad dressings, fast foods, and restaurant meals.

For clarity's sake, high-quality healthy fats and sources of fat include:

- Olives and olive oil (Make sure it's third party–certified as pure; 80 percent of olive oils are adulterated with vegetable oils. Also avoid cooking with olive oil, as it becomes oxidized at a low heat threshold. Instead, use it cold.)

- Coconuts and coconut oil (excellent for cooking, as it can withstand higher temperatures without oxidizing)

- Avocados

- Organic grass-fed meats

- Organic pastured egg yolks

- Animal-based omega-3 fat, such as krill oil, and small fatty fish like sardines and anchovies

- Butter and ghee (clarified butter) made from raw, grass-fed, organic milk

- Organic raw nuts that are high in fat with only moderate amounts of protein, such as macadamias and pecans

- MCT oil, which is derived from coconut oil; the "MCT" stands for medium-chain triglyceride

- Organic seeds like black sesame, cumin, pumpkin, and hemp

- Raw cacao butter

- Chicken and duck fat (excellent for cooking)

- Lard and tallow (also great for cooking)

It's important to maximize the quality of the protein. Look to raw organic nuts and seeds and organic and pastured eggs and meats for your primary sources of high-quality protein.

To nudge your body into the fat-burning zone, restrict your net carbs—which, as I said, is the total grams of carbs minus the grams of fiber—to less than 20 to 50 grams per day. And keep your protein to less than 1 gram per kilogram of lean body mass, which for most people will come to 30 to 60 grams.

KEEP TRACK OF YOUR CARBS

It is likely you do not know how to measure net carbs, which is why it is important (at least initially) to obtain an electronic digital scale and get an account at Cronometer.com/mercola so you can precisely know how many grams of net carbs and protein you are actually eating. It is typically best to enter your foods before you eat them so you can modify your food choices to achieve your goals.

Cronometer will help you track exactly how many grams of net carbs, fats, and protein you eat. It will make all the calculations for you—based on the parameters you enter such as your height, weight, body fat percentage, and waist circumference—to show you how you are doing on hitting your macronutrient targets. It really is so informative and inspiring to see the quantitative breakdown of the food you're eating. The only hitch is that to get the most out of Cronometer, you really need to log every bit of food that you eat as accurately as possible, which typically requires weighing your food. You can, however, enter the foods that you eat frequently so you can easily select them from a drop-down menu instead of manually entering them each time. You can even download Cronometer to your smartphone and easily update your food logs when you're on the go.

When You Eat Matters Too

When it comes to teaching your body to burn fat instead of glucose as its primary fuel, it's not just what you eat that matters—it's when you eat it too. By compressing your mealtimes into a window of just six to eight hours, you initiate a number of beneficial processes in the body that promote fat-burning and weight loss. This approach is known as intermittent fasting, and it's a powerful complement to a ketogenic diet.

I realize that suggesting that you eat during a smaller window of time during the day goes against conventional wisdom, which says it's important to have three meals—plus up to two snacks—per day, or that you should have a snack before bedtime to promote sleep. In addition, the fast-food industry has made high-carb, high-calorie food ridiculously accessible. Yet, if regularly going without food were detrimental to human health, we would never have survived and flourished as a species. Your body has evolved to not only survive even when food isn't available, but also to *thrive* despite food scarcity. For all the attention that we pay to eating and the role it plays in weight and health, we owe it to ourselves to also examine the flip side of that coin: not eating.

So far, research overwhelmingly supports this notion that ditching the three-square-meals-a-day approach in favor of intermittent fasting may do wonders for your health.

Science has proven that fasting yields the following benefits:

- Helps promote insulin sensitivity

- Normalizes levels of ghrelin, also known as the "hunger hormone"

- Increases the rate of human growth hormone production, which has an important role in health, fitness, and slowing the aging process

- Lowers triglyceride levels

- Helps suppress inflammation and fight free radical damage

While I used to recommend skipping breakfast and making lunch your first meal, I eventually learned that for most, skipping dinner is a far more effective strategy. However you choose to fast, be sure to have your last bite of food at least three hours before you go to bed. This is because your least metabolically active state is while you are sleeping, so the last thing you want to do is add fuel you don't need in the evening. Doing so will simply generate excess dangerous free radicals.

Eating only during a six- to eight-hour window each day can take a few weeks to adapt to and should be done gradually. Once your body has shifted into fat-burning mode, it will be easier for you to fast for as long as 18 hours and still feel satiated. Your craving for sugar will slowly dissipate, and managing your weight will be easier.

As powerful as it is, intermittent fasting is not something you should carelessly undertake. *Always* pay close attention to your body and your energy level. If you are hypoglycemic or diabetic, you should avoid any type of calorie restriction until your blood sugar or insulin levels are regulated. Fasting is not recommended if you are pregnant or breast-feeding.

One note of caution: It is not advisable to practice intermittent fasting if your daily diet is filled with processed foods. Addressing the quality of your diet is crucial before you venture into fasting. Within the six to eight hours that you do eat, you need to eliminate refined carbohydrates like pizza, bread, and potatoes and fill your diet with high-fiber vegetables, healthy protein, and healthy fats such as butter, eggs, avocado, coconut oil, olive oil, and raw nuts.

THE SURPRISING BENEFITS OF FASTING

It is helpful to think about fasting as a beneficial stressor. Much as exercise cues your body to grow stronger, fasting initiates metabolic processes that promote overall health, including:

- **Reduced blood sugar.** In the absence of food, blood glucose levels fall, typically to well below 100.

- **Lowered levels of insulin and improved insulin resistance.** As a result of lower blood glucose levels, less insulin is released because there is no need to move glucose out of the bloodstream. With less insulin in circulation, insulin receptor sites get a chance to recalibrate and heal, reducing insulin resistance as well.

- **A rejuvenated gut and immune system.** With no food to break down, the digestive tract gets some time off to rest and recuperate. And since 80 percent of your immune system is in the gut, it gets a break too, enabling it to focus instead on regenerating the body's organs.

- **Boosted ketone production.** Ketones prevent your liver from breaking down your body's own tissue in the absence of food, preserving muscle mass. They also provide a needed alternative to glucose for the brain and central nervous system.

- **Increased metabolic rate.** In the absence of food, your body raises its level of adrenaline to provide energy. As a result, your overall metabolic rate increases. This is contrary to popular belief that fasting slows metabolism by putting it into "starvation mode."

- **Improved detoxification.** A side effect of fasting is increased autophagy—the process by which your body recycles damaged cells and sweeps away toxins and other cellular debris. This crucial process reduces inflammation, slows the growth of cancer cells, and slows aging.

- **Reduced hunger.** As your insulin and leptin levels lower, so does your appetite. You may need to adapt to burning fat before you experience this benefit, a process that can take anywhere from a couple of days to a couple of months. But once you achieve it, you will be freed from constant craving and appetite.

- **Lowered body fat.** Because it encourages your body to burn fat for fuel, fasting leads to reduced fat stores.

- **Reduced levels of hormones thought to promote cancer.** Fasting reduces levels of insulin-like growth factor 1 (IGF-1), a hormone that induces cell growth and replication. While some IGF-1 is beneficial, in excess amounts it is associated with cancer, which is essentially the growth of cells run rampant.

- **Protected brain function.** Fasting also appears to prevent degeneration of brain cells.

With all these powerful benefits, it's no wonder that intermittent fasting is becoming more and more popular, even receiving coverage in such mainstream magazines as *Vogue*.

CONTRAINDICATIONS FOR FASTING

As much as I believe in the power of intermittent fasting, it isn't suitable for everyone. If you have any of the following diseases, fast only with medical supervision:

- Diabetes
- Adrenal challenges
- Chronic renal disease
- Cancer
- Cortisol dysregulation
- Anorexia nervosa or bulimia

If you have a disease called porphyria, are pregnant or nursing, are malnourished or underweight, or are under 18, you should not fast.

Everyone who undertakes intermittent fasting should be on the lookout for signs of low blood sugar, including:

- Lightheadedness
- Shakiness
- Confusion
- Fainting
- Excessive sweating
- Blurred vision
- Slurred speech
- Feelings of an atypical heartbeat

- Pins-and-needles sensation in the fingertips

If you experience any of these symptoms, eat something that will not raise your blood sugar, such as coconut oil dissolved in a cup of black coffee or tea.

A KETOGENIC DIET + INTERMITTENT FASTING = MITOCHONDRIAL METABOLIC THERAPY

I call the combination of a ketogenic diet and intermittent fasting Mitochondrial Metabolic Therapy (MMT). Together, they have incredible power to boost your health by optimizing your mitochondrial function and protecting your mitochondria from potential damage that could lead to disease.

While MMT is quite a paradigm shift from the typical diet advice you'll find in mainstream media and Western medicine, as you embark on it you will quickly find that it is also a delicious and satisfying way to eat. By experimenting with the recipes that Pete has so expertly created for us and incorporating them into your daily regimen, you will see that it is possible to feel radiantly healthy and effortlessly find and maintain an ideal weight without any sense of deprivation. MMT is an eating plan, but it is so much more than a diet. It's a path to health and a way of life.

REV UP YOUR DIGESTION

Countless books have been written about digestion, yet the science—and therefore our understanding—of how your body breaks down and utilizes nutrients is still in its infancy. This section is a mere overview of what we know to be accurate at the time of this writing: the physical processes at work in the act of digestion, some possible causes of imbalance in your digestive system, and what to do if it does become unbalanced.

What is digestion exactly? The short answer is that it is the act of breaking down the food or liquid you consume into constituents of a size that your body can use as fuel or a structural component for your body.

Fairly basic, right? And yet, digestion is actually a complex combination of biological interactions and chemical reactions taking place at every stop along the extensive digestive tract, which is generally split into two halves—the upper gastrointestinal tract (mouth, esophagus, stomach, and duodenum) and the lower gastrointestinal tract (small intestine and large intestine).

Your gastrointestinal tract is also home to the largest part of your body's immune system, protecting you against foreign invaders by producing acids and housing colonies of beneficial bacteria that act as a defensive army fighting to protect you from pathogens that find their way inside your body.

Once you select something to eat, your mouth goes to work, using your tongue and teeth to turn large pieces of food into smaller pieces (mastication) and using enzymes from your salivary glands to begin chemically breaking down food into molecules that your body can absorb.

This is why nutrition experts are always advising you to eat slowly and chew your food thoroughly (at least 20 chews per bite): because your digestion actually begins in your mouth! Taking your time when eating and chewing your food properly has a number of beneficial side effects. For example, chewing your food twice as long as you normally would will help you control your portion sizes, which naturally decreases calorie consumption.

Another benefit of chewing longer is that your food is digested better. The majority of your digestive enzymes are actually in your mouth, not in your stomach. Therefore, chewing your food longer allows the food to be broken down better. You're also likely to find that you actually enjoy the *taste* of the food more if you eat more slowly. Additionally, chewing your food helps stimulate the production of enzymes to help digest it.

Also, the first major *problem* with digestion starts with what you choose to put in your mouth! Clearly, though, because you have picked up this book, you are dedicated to choosing healthy, natural, whole foods rather than the plethora of processed so-called foods available on the market today. You're doing yourself and your health a powerful favor by doing so.

WHAT GOES ON WHEN FOOD REACHES YOUR STOMACH

Moving down your digestive tract, once food is swallowed, it travels down your esophagus and enters your stomach. The environment inside your stomach is highly acidic (pH 4), and this acid—composed of hydrochloric acid and pepsin—acts as a defense mechanism against harmful pathogens that might have slipped in with your food. A protective mucous lining protects your stomach tissues from all this acid.

When you are young, your body usually will produce sufficient acid to properly digest your food, but as you age, reduced stomach acid comes along with the territory. This explains why, as you get older, it is common to experience heartburn, indigestion, and conditions associated with gastroesophageal reflux disease (GERD). Contrary to what you may think, unpleasant symptoms associated with acid reflux and heartburn are typically caused by a *reduction* in stomach acid, not the overproduction of it. This is news to many, because the drug companies spend loads of marketing money to convince you that too much stomach acid is the problem and their drugs are the simple solution.

Digestive aids like hydrochloric acid (HCL), enzymes, and probiotics can actually be highly effective tools to maintain a more acidic and beneficial environment in your stomach and intestines, helping your digestive system work optimally.

Moving further along, after leaving the stomach your food enters the small intestine. Recent estimates suggest that there are about 30 trillion microorganisms living in your gut.[1] These tiny creatures make up three to five pounds of your body weight!

These microorganisms—bacteria, yeasts, and fungi—help your body break down foods into their component parts. They can produce beneficial waste products as they feast on your digesting food, such as B and K vitamins. They are also able to break down some foods that your body cannot absorb by itself. For example, they change carbs into simple sugars and proteins into their component amino acids.

But not all intestinal organisms are helpful. This is yet another way that the food you eat impacts your health. Some foods, like the indigestible fiber in vegetables, are metabolized to short-chain fatty acids in your gut, which nurture good bacteria and starve the bad. But some foods, like processed foods and sugar, have the opposite effect.

One of the best things you can do for your health, including your digestive health, is eliminate sugars and processed foods as much as possible! In doing so, you can avoid being one of the millions of people who currently suffer from disease-causing organisms like yeast overgrowth.

Estimates are that as many as 80 million people, mostly women, are currently suffering from harmful yeast overgrowth. Symptoms include:

- Irritable bowel syndrome
- Migraines

- PMS
- Cancer
- Vaginitis
- Asthma
- Fibromyalgia
- Weight gain
- Food allergies
- Chronic fatigue
- Vaginal or oral (thrush) yeast infections
- Depression

The key to good intestinal health, especially in your small intestine, is maintaining the ideal balance of helpful and harmful microorganisms. (You may be wondering, why would anyone want *any* harmful microbes? The fact is, they are part of life and impossible to completely eradicate. So long as you have plenty of friendly bacteria to keep them in check, they aren't likely to negatively impact your health.) The approach to eating that I outline in my book *Fat for Fuel*, and that the recipes in this book follow, is a powerful way to do just that.

Other symptoms you may face if your gut microorganisms are out of balance for long periods of time include:

- Bad breath
- Flatulence
- Toxemia
- Chronic fatigue
- Mental fogginess
- Decreased immunity

- Impaired digestion and absorption

Nowadays, it truly does take an act of will to train your body to recognize whole natural foods as delicious and nutritious, when the alternative is food-like substances that have been processed, designed, crafted, and marketed to appeal to all of your senses and to your intellect.

If you love the convenience and taste of packaged foods, don't despair. Once you start cooking and enjoying the recipes included in this book that are based on the whole-foods, low-carb, high-fat approach, you'll quickly see that eating healthy isn't an act of deprivation. Quite the opposite—as the body starts burning fat as its primary fuel, most people notice that their cravings actually disappear.

Additionally, real foods are so delicious and energizing (and the high-quality fats so satiating) that you will soon stop thinking about the processed stuff. Your taste buds as well as your beneficial bacteria will thank you.

WHEN DIGESTION STARTS EATING YOU UP: LEAKY GUT SYNDROME

The lining of your gut is very thin, only one cell thick, and it is quite easy and very common for disruptions in the cellular connections to occur. When there's a disruption in the interconnections between the cells in your intestines, this allows undigested food particles to enter your bloodstream. This is known as leaky gut syndrome, a serious problem that can contribute to an autoimmune response.

If your gut lining is leaky or permeable, partially undigested food, toxins, viruses, yeast, and bacteria have the opportunity to pass through your intestine and access your bloodstream. When your intestinal lining is repeatedly damaged due to reoccurring leaky gut, cells called microvilli become damaged and unable to process and utilize the nutrients and enzymes that are vital to proper digestion.

Eventually, digestion is impaired and absorption of nutrients is negatively affected. As more exposure occurs, your body initiates an attack on these foreign invaders leaking from the gut. It responds with inflammation, allergic reactions, and other symptoms we associate with a variety of diseases.

Leaky gut is the root of many allergies and autoimmune disorders. Combine it with toxic overload and you have a perfect storm that can lead to neurological disorders like autism, ADHD, and learning disabilities.

NOURISH YOUR INTESTINAL FLORA TO RESTORE GUT HEALTH

Keeping your population of favorable intestinal bacteria healthy is the key to optimizing your digestive well-being, but the benefits don't end there. These organisms perform a wide variety of vital functions, and we've now come to realize that they need to be properly balanced and nourished if we want to maintain multiple facets of physical as well as mental health.

Researchers are now realizing that *your microbiome* may be among the most important factors in preventing as many as 90 percent

of diseases. We used to think that DNA was the most important factor in disease development, but now we know that while genes do play a role, the actual expression of their code is in large part regulated by which microbes are present! Emerging science also shows that your microbiome can be rapidly altered, for better or worse, by factors such as diet, lifestyle, and chemical exposures.

This is a double-edged sword, no doubt. On the one hand, many of our modern conveniences (such as processed foods, antibiotics, chlorinated water, and pesticides) turn out to be extremely detrimental to our gut flora. On the other hand, your diet is one of the easiest, fastest, and most effective ways to improve and optimize your microbiome. So the good news is that you have a great degree of control over your health destiny.

Bacteria appear to influence human health in two important ways. While an overabundance of pathogenic (disease-causing) bacteria has been linked to various diseases, other microbes appear to be actively involved in preventing certain disease states. When they're lacking, you end up losing this protection, which allows the disease process to set in.

Studies have linked certain bacteria to several diseases, including obesity.[2] This in no way changes the fact that certain foods will make you pack on the pounds; it just means that the bacteria these foods nourish likely play a major role in facilitating that process. The foods known to produce metabolic dysfunction and insulin resistance (such as processed foods, fructose/sugar, and artificial sweeteners) also severely impair your beneficial gut bacteria, and this may well be a key mechanism by which these foods promote obesity.

Chemicals may also contribute to a weight problem by way of the gut microbiome. For example, a study published in *Environmental Health Perspectives* found that persistent organic pollutants (POPs) found in food altered the gut microbiome in mice, thereby contributing to the development of obesity and metabolic dysfunction.[3] Conversely, another study found that one microbe called *Akkermansia muciniphila* helps ward off obesity, diabetes, and heart disease by lowering blood sugar, improving insulin resistance, and promoting a healthier distribution of body fat.[4] However, it's still not known whether *A. muciniphila* produces these effects all on its own, or whether it helps promote other beneficial bacteria.

Research has also shown that gut microbes specializing in fermenting soluble fiber play an important role in preventing inflammatory disorders, as they help calibrate your immune system.[5] The inflammatory response actually starts in your gut and then travels to your brain, which subsequently sends signals to the rest of your body in a complex feedback loop. So in order to address chronic inflammation and inflammatory diseases, it's important to nourish your gut flora.

Researchers have also linked diets high in processed sugar to memory and learning impairments, courtesy of altered gut bacteria.[6] Impairments in your microbiome not only promote neurological diseases but can also have a powerful impact on your general mood. Depression is increasingly being viewed as a symptom of poor gut health, and therein may lie the real cure as well.

For example, in one recent study researchers found that fermented foods and drinks helped curb social anxiety disorder in young adults.[7] Previous trials have also demonstrated that probiotics can help ease both anxiety and depression. For example, one study found that in certain brain regions, the probiotic *Lactobacillus rhamnosus* had a marked effect on levels of GABA, an inhibitory neurotransmitter that is significantly involved in regulating many physiological and psychological processes.[8] It also lowered the stress-induced hormone corticosterone, resulting in reduced anxiety- and depression-related behavior.

In another study, people who took a multi-strain probiotic for at least four weeks reported a lessening of rumination—recurring, persistent thoughts about something distressing that has happened or may happen, which tends to create anxiety.[9]

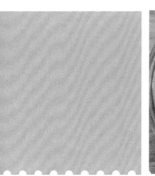
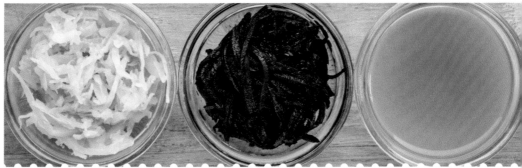

BEWARE OF "PROBIOTIC" JUNK FOOD— PARTICULARLY YOGURT

Because the news is out about the beneficial impact of probiotics, there are many food products on the market that claim to be good sources of beneficial bacteria. One of the most popular is yogurt. But most commercially available yogurts are nothing more than creamy junk food.

Commercial yogurts often contain upwards of 25 to 30 grams of sugar per serving, which meets or exceeds the recommended amount of sugar *for the whole day*! The amount of probiotics you'll get from commercial yogurt is also far lower than what you'd get from a high-quality probiotic supplement. A commercial yogurt might give you a million probiotic cells, which sounds like a lot, but if you take a quality supplement you're getting *tens of billions* of probiotics—four orders of magnitude greater amounts. So in that respect, a supplement is clearly easier and more cost-effective. Another option is to make yogurt at home.

To find out how your favorite brand of yogurt rates, use the Cornucopia Institute's Yogurt Buyer's Guide and Scorecard, which is available at http://cornucopia.org/yogurt-scorecard/.

OPTIMIZING YOUR MICROBIOME IS A POTENT DISEASE-PREVENTION STRATEGY

You will be pleased to know that supporting your microbiome isn't very complicated. However, you do need to take proactive steps to implement certain key strategies while actively avoiding other factors. To optimize your microbiome both inside and out, consider the following recommendations:

- Eat plenty of fermented foods to continually repopulate your friendly bacterial population.

- Take a high-quality, multi-strain probiotic supplement, which I will cover in detail a little later.

- Boost your soluble and insoluble fiber intake, focusing on non-starchy vegetables, nuts, and seeds, including sprouted seeds. The recipes in this book will help you do exactly that.

- Get your hands dirty in the garden. Lack of exposure to the outdoors can in and of itself cause your microbiome to become deficient.[10] Garden work can help reacquaint your immune system with beneficial microorganisms on the plants and in the soil.

- Open your windows. Research shows that opening a window and increasing natural airflow can improve the diversity and health of the microbes in your home, which in turn benefits you.[11]

- Wash your dishes by hand instead of in the dishwasher. This leaves more bacteria on the dishes than dishwashers do, and eating off these less-than-sterile dishes can actually nurture your microbiome.

- Avoid antibiotics, unless absolutely necessary, as they don't discriminate between harmful and friendly bacteria. And when you do need to take antibiotics, make sure to reseed your gut with fermented foods and/or a probiotic supplement. Because the antibiotic is liable to simply kill the friendly bacteria contained in the probiotic supplement if you take them both at the same time, take your probiotic a few hours before or after taking the antibiotic.

- Switch from conventionally raised meats and dairy to pastured, organic versions. Animals raised on feedlots are routinely fed low-dose antibiotics and genetically engineered grains loaded with the herbicide glyphosate (the main ingredient in Roundup), which is widely known to kill many bacteria.

- Filter your drinking and bathing water. Commonly added chemicals including chlorine and disinfection by-products can be harmful to your friendly bacteria.

- Eat organic produce, since many agricultural chemicals, in particular glyphosate, will actively kill many of your beneficial gut microbes.

- Steer clear of antibacterial soap, which kills off both good and bad bacteria.

THE ROLE OF PROBIOTIC SUPPLEMENTS IN GUT HEALTH

One of the best and least expensive ways to optimize your gut microbiome is to change your diet by eliminating sugars and processed foods and eating real food, preferably organic, including plenty of fiber and traditionally fermented foods. But probiotics can also be beneficial.

Probiotics are supplements designed to increase the population of beneficial bacteria in your gut. You might imagine that you need to take the supplements for only a little while and then the bacteria grow, reproduce, and live happily after. But that's actually not the case. Your intestinal tract is a challenging environment with lots of competition. Probiotics have developed the ability to withstand a lot of difficult conditions, including stomach acid and bile, but they don't live and thrive forever.

Rather, when you stop taking probiotics, your populations of friendly bacteria will gradually decline. So it's really important to continue consuming probiotics. If you can't commit to eating fermented foods—particularly vegetables—regularly, probiotic supplements are a good alternative.

Not all probiotic supplements are created equal, however. You'll need to choose your supplement well. Factors to consider include the following:

- Pick a reputable brand. If you trust the products made by a company, perhaps it's doing a great job making probiotics as well.

- Look for a potency count of 50 billion colony-forming units (CFUs) or higher. That's the number of bacteria being delivered per dose.

- Assess shelf life. Avoid capsules that only tell you the CFUs *at time of manufacture*. You want to know that the bacteria will still be alive when you actually swallow the capsule.

- Favor brands that include multiple species of bacteria, as high diversity of bacterial strains tends to be associated with better health. That said, products containing species of *Lactobacillus* and *Bifidobacteria* are generally recommended.

- Look for non-GMO brands, and confirm that they adhere to Current Good Manufacturing Practices (CGMPs), a pharmaceutical guideline established and maintained by the U.S. Food and Drug Administration (FDA).

I hope you're coming to see that nurturing your digestion through dietary choices has powerful and wide-ranging effects on numerous aspects of your health. Eating clean and natural foods, nourishing your gut, and having a healthy intestinal community are really at the core of wellness.

TAKE AIM AT DIABETES

In the United States, 115 million people—or nearly one in three—have some form of diabetes or pre-diabetes.[1] Of these people, 86 million have pre-diabetes, a condition in which blood sugar levels are higher than normal (about 100 to 125 milligrams per deciliter in a fasting state), but not yet high enough to be diagnosed as full-blown diabetes. And of these 86 million, 15 to 30 percent will go on to develop type 2 diabetes in the next five years.

Type 2 diabetes isn't the only disease associated with pre-diabetes—a meta-analysis that included data from more than 900,000 people found that those with pre-diabetes have a 15 percent higher risk of developing cancer, particularly cancers of the liver, stomach, pancreas, breast, or endometrium.[2]

Why is diabetes becoming so prevalent? Because of our overconsumption of sugars, starches, and processed foods, which leads to high blood sugar levels, high insulin levels, insulin resistance, and being overweight (although you certainly can have type 2 diabetes without being overweight). An additional result is the inability to burn fat as your primary fuel, which keeps you stuck in an unhealthy loop.

The often-overlooked good news here is that type 2 diabetes is completely preventable and nearly 100 percent treatable—when you address the root cause, that is. Sadly, this is not the approach of most conventionally trained physicians.

Chances are, if your blood glucose levels are elevated and you consult with your doctor about it, you'll be checked for diabetes, and there is a great chance you will be put on an oral hypoglycemic drug or even worse, insulin.

Your doctor will say that the purpose of taking these shots or pills is to lower your blood sugar. She may even explain to you that this is necessary because insulin regulation plays such an integral role in your health and longevity. The doctor might add that elevated glucose levels are symptoms not only of diabetes, but also of heart disease, peripheral vascular disease, stroke, high blood pressure, cancer, and obesity. And she would be correct in all of that.

But would she go beyond that explanation to tell you what part insulin and leptin play in this process, or that when your body develops a resistance to leptin, you're on your way to diabetes, if you're not already there?

Probably not.

Conventional medicine has type 2 diabetes pegged as a problem with blood sugar control, but this is simply a superficial and deeply flawed understanding. The reality is that diabetes is a disease rooted in *insulin resistance*, which occurs when, as I discussed in Chapter 1, you have plenty of insulin circulating in your blood, to the point that insulin receptors become desensitized to it.

When this happens, your cells become resistant to insulin, which, as you'll recall, is a hormone secreted by your pancreas that normalizes sugar levels in your blood. So when you are insulin resistant, your blood sugar levels tend to rise.

Those rising blood sugar levels can then trigger a disruption of leptin signaling. As I discussed in Chapter 1, leptin is a hormone produced by your fat cells that tells your brain you have enough fat stored and that you have eaten enough. It's also involved in your immune system, your reproductive system, and regulating how much energy you burn.

There's one more hormone that's intimately involved with diabetes, and that is ghrelin. This hormone is secreted by your stomach lining and tells your brain that you're hungry.

With a malfunction of leptin or ghrelin signaling, you may eat too much food for your activity level and rate of metabolism, resulting in weight gain and obesity. With obesity often comes a resistance to insulin, resulting in high blood sugar and a diagnosis of diabetes.

You can thank researchers Jeffrey M. Friedman and Douglas Coleman for discovering leptin and its role in the body in 1994. Interestingly, Friedman based its name on the Greek word *leptos*, which means "thin," after he discovered that mice injected with synthetic leptin became more active and lost weight.

But when Friedman also found that obese people have very high levels of leptin in their blood, he realized that something else must be going on. And that "something" was that obesity can cause a resistance to leptin. Friedman and Coleman also discovered that leptin is responsible for the accuracy of insulin signaling and for your insulin resistance.

This is why "treating" diabetes by merely concentrating on lowering blood sugar and using drugs or insulin can be a dangerous approach. It simply does not address the foundational cause, which is metabolic miscommunication that's going on in every cell of your body when you have insulin and leptin resistance.

Taking insulin results in even greater danger to type 2 diabetes patients, as it worsens their leptin and insulin resistance over time. The only known way to reestablish proper leptin (and insulin) signaling is through teaching your body to burn fat as your primary fuel. And I promise, your diet can have a more profound influence on your health than any known drug or modality of medical treatment.

When you bring your blood glucose levels down over the long term by adopting the low-carb, adequate-protein, and quality high-fat formula that the recipes in this book follow, you create the conditions for lipase (a pancreatic enzyme that breaks down fat) to be activated; ghrelin, leptin, and insulin levels to normalize; leptin and insulin resistance to resolve, and pre-diabetes and type 2 diabetes to be reversed.

To be sure that you're helping all these important things happen, you'll want to start measuring and tracking your blood glucose levels throughout the day so you can be sure it is indeed coming down over time.

MONITORING YOUR BLOOD SUGAR LEVELS

Knowing your blood sugar level helps you understand precisely how your body is working. The wonderful aspect of this is that you don't have to go to the doctor; you can do it in the convenience of your own home and for less than 25 cents a reading. This is largely due to the tens of millions of diabetics that have driven the cost of this test way down.

Please don't become intimidated by this process. Remember, tens of millions of diabetics do this every day. By finding your blood sugar, you will have a powerful tool to help you burn fat for fuel. It will also insulate you from ever developing diabetes and having to regularly do this test for the rest of your life.

Initially you will test your blood glucose levels twice a day:

- When you first wake up, before eating anything, to establish a baseline for the day.

- Just before you go to bed, to evaluate the impact of your food choices on your blood sugar that day.

But remember that this is only until you are able to burn fat for fuel. Once you achieve this metabolic flexibility, you will not need to test yourself unless you get off the program or are curious.

Seeing your blood glucose numbers will give you real-time insight into how your food choices affect your blood sugar; accordingly, regularly testing your levels will help motivate you to continue to choose foods that fit the low-carb, moderate-protein, high-fat model, as these types of food will help bring your readings down over time.

When you first start eating this way, you can expect to see your glucose numbers jump around quite a bit—rather than get alarmed by an unexpectedly high number, focus on the trend over a couple of weeks and months. You'll know you're on the right track when you can see your numbers trend downward and become more stable. This means that your pancreas isn't having to work so hard to produce so much insulin, and that your insulin receptors will get a chance to regain their sensitivity since there won't be so much insulin floating around anymore.

In order to test your blood glucose, you'll need to buy a few items:

- A glucose monitor. Most glucose meters range from $7 to $50, and they are often discounted or free with coupons. I prefer the Bayer Contour—the monitor is under $10 and the test strips are only 25 cents each. The Bayer Contour Next is newer, but I found the older model to be more reliable when I tested them.

- Glucose test strips. These retail for as little as 25 cents and as much as $2 a strip. Since you'll be testing two times a day and using a new strip each time, these can get expensive, so I recommend going with one of the cheaper options.

- Lancets. You use these micro-sized needles to prick your finger for the drop of blood you need to apply to the test strip. They are inexpensive and easy to find.

- A lancet-holding device. This administers the pinprick of the lancet.

Because there are so many people with diabetes in the United States, all these supplies are readily (and inexpensively) available on Amazon or at your local drugstore or discount department store (such as Target or Wal-Mart) without a prescription.

Once you get your readings, you'll want to record them somewhere. If you prefer paper and pencil, keep them in a notebook or jot them down on a calendar. I recommend logging them into the online diet and health tracking tool Cronometer.com, which I cover in more detail in Chapter 5. Whichever method you choose, seeing your numbers trend downward over time is incredibly gratifying and motivating.

You'll also want to monitor your fasting insulin level, which is every bit as important as your fasting blood sugar. Although you need a blood test from a doctor's office to do it, the information it gives you about your insulin sensitivity is worth the hassle. Your fasting insulin level should be less than 4. The higher your level, the worse your insulin sensitivity is.

ADDRESS YOUR DIET

As I mentioned earlier, most of the food people eat these days skews metabolism toward insulin resistance and type 2 diabetes. Most Americans are burning glucose as their primary fuel, which elevates blood sugar, promotes insulin resistance, and inhibits your body's ability to access and burn body fat—hence, the connection between obesity and diabetes.

Healthy fat, meanwhile, is a far preferable sort of fuel, as it burns much more efficiently than carbs. One of the most important dietary recommendations is to limit net carbs (total carbohydrates minus fiber) and protein, replacing them with higher amounts of high-quality, healthy fats. A key way of preventing diabetes is to keep your net carbs below 50 grams per day.

Keep in mind that the only way you'll know how many total carbs, fiber, and net carbs you eat is to accurately measure them. The simplest way of doing this is to use an online nutrition tracker and to weigh your food with an inexpensive electronic digital kitchen scale (see page 9 and pages 48–49 to learn more about my favorite online food tracker, Cronometer.com).

Another important component is to boost your fiber intake considerably. Research shows that people with high intakes of dietary fiber have a significantly lower risk of obesity and diabetes.[3] Aim for at least 50 grams of fiber per day. Foods that are particularly good sources of fiber include almonds, berries (eat only a handful to keep net-carb consumption down), broccoli, brussels sprouts, cauliflower, chia seeds, flax seeds (ground), green beans, hemp seeds, and psyllium seed husk. I discuss fiber intake in more detail on page 41.

ADDITIONAL WAYS TO CONTROL BLOOD SUGAR, NATURALLY

Although changing your diet is the most powerful way to treat pre-diabetes and type 2 diabetes, there are many other approaches that will support your efforts and help you reap even greater health rewards:

- **Exercise.** The more you exercise, the more your cells will be sensitive to leptin. And greater sensitivity to leptin reduces your potential resistance to insulin and therefore your risk of diabetes.[4]

- **Reduce stress.** When you become stressed, your body secretes cortisol and glucagon, both of which affect your blood sugar level.[5,6] Control your stress using exercise, meditation, yoga, prayer, or other relaxation techniques that appeal to you.

- **Sleep.** Getting enough quality sleep is necessary to feel well and experience good health. Poor sleeping habits may reduce insulin sensitivity and promote weight gain.[7]

- **Take vitamin D.** Have you been getting adequate sun exposure? Studies done within the past decade strongly suggest that vitamin D is highly beneficial in addressing type 2 diabetes.[8,9] Other studies, published between 1990 and 2009,[10] also revealed a significant link between high levels of vitamin D and a lowered risk of developing type 2 diabetes, along with cardiovascular disease and metabolic syndrome. To optimize your vitamin D levels, regularly expose a large amount of your skin to healthy amounts of sunshine, preferably as close to solar noon as possible. Direct UV exposure translates to up to 20,000 units of vitamin D a day. You may also supplement with oral vitamin D3. If you choose to do the latter, have your vitamin D level (25 hydroxy D) routinely tested by a proficient lab to make sure it is in the 40–60 ng/ml range.

IN SUMMARY

Type 2 diabetes is a fully preventable, reversible condition that arises from faulty leptin signaling and insulin resistance. It is possible to control or reverse your diabetes without drugs by recovering your insulin and leptin sensitivities. The only known way to reestablish proper leptin and insulin signaling is through proper diet and exercise. There is NO drug that can currently accomplish this, and I doubt that one will ever exist in the lifetime of anyone reading this!

The good news is that you don't have to be a part of the diabetes epidemic. The tips, recipes, and dietary guidelines included in this book can help you avoid becoming a dismal statistic!

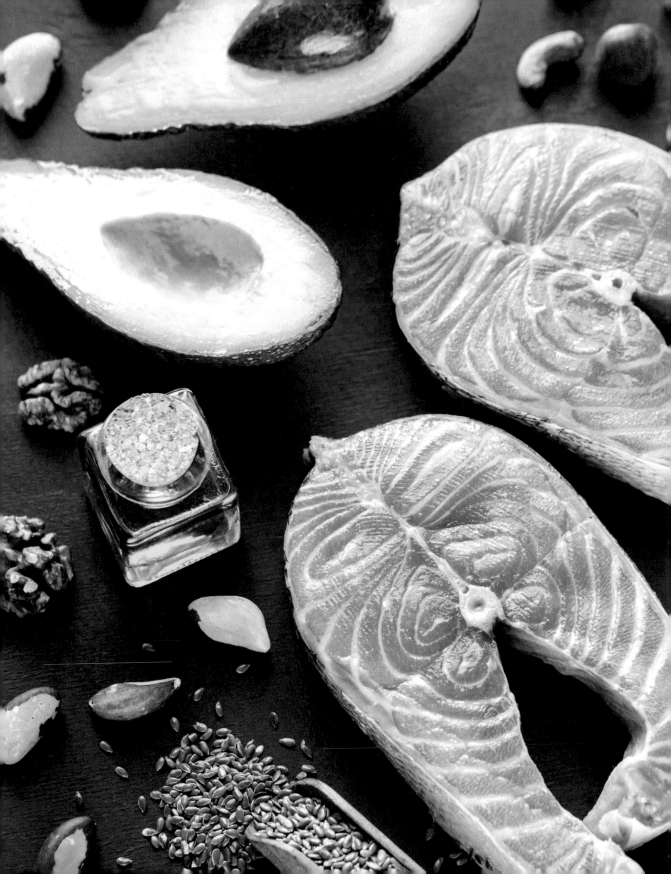

REGULATE YOUR WEIGHT

In the United States, about 75 percent of men and 67 percent of women are now either overweight (with a Body Mass Index, a calculation of your weight in kilograms divided by the square of your height in meters, also known as BMI, over 25) or obese (a BMI over 30)—that's three out of four men and two out of three women. This has risen significantly from figures gathered between 1988 and 1994, when "just" 63 percent of American men and 55 percent of American women were overweight or obese.[1]

Environmental and lifestyle factors—such as hormone-disrupting chemicals used in the food supply and in consumer products, a growing lack of basic physical activity, poor sleep habits, and stress—play a significant role in this trend, which is why you have to incorporate some lifestyle strategies that enhance health, such as yoga. For now, though, I want to focus on the trends in food and eating that have contributed to the obesity epidemic, so you can start making wiser choices right away. They are, in no particular order:

- **Highly processed and genetically engineered (GE) foods.** These primary culprits are chock-full of ingredients that both individually and in combination contribute to metabolic dysfunction and hard-to-control weight gain.

- **Aggressive marketing of harmful junk food.** Marketing makes these highly processed and GE foods seem irresistible and ubiquitous. The siren call of convenience, too, is hard to resist for a population that feels more and more strapped for time.

- **Food policy.** Farmers are incentivized to grow ever more GE corn syrup, GE vegetable oils, and GE sugar to the point that these ingredients are now foundational in the U.S. diet and are increasingly found worldwide. Wherever a highly processed diet becomes the norm, obesity inevitably follows.

But perhaps the biggest contributing factor to rising obesity rates is the low-fat craze.

THE TRUTH ABOUT FAT

Most conventional physicians, nutritionists, and public health experts have long claimed that dietary fat promotes heart disease and obesity, due in large part to a misinformation campaign based on faulty research that began in the mid-20th century (see my book *Fat for Fuel* for a deeper dive into this subject). This deception has caused people to follow conventional low-fat, high-carb diets, which has ruined the health of millions.

For the past five decades, many people have turned away from healthy fats like butter, eggs, and full-fat dairy and shifted to whole grains and cereals instead. This is in response to conventional wisdom to eat a diet high in complex carbohydrates and low in saturated fat.

However, many recent studies have found that replacing saturated fats with carbohydrates actually leads to detrimental cardiometabolic consequences, as well as increased risk of obesity, inflammation, heart disease, and cancer. Research has consistently demonstrated that low-fat diets do not prevent heart disease. It's actually industrially processed and heated vegetable oils loaded with trans fat and cyclic aldehydes—not saturated fat and healthy dietary cholesterol—that clog your arteries.[2] Trans fats and other toxic metabolites in heated, processed vegetable oils also interfere with your insulin receptors, thereby increasing your risk for diabetes and related health problems.[3]

Overindulging in sugar and grains overwhelms your brain too. Having consistently high levels of glucose and insulin blunts its insulin signaling, which can lead to impaired thinking and memory, eventually contributing to permanent brain damage and playing a key role in diseases like Alzheimer's (which has even been dubbed "type 3 diabetes").

All these reasons make trading healthy, unprocessed saturated fats for added sugars and industrially processed vegetable oils among the worst lifestyle alterations to occur in modern history.

Not only are saturated fats essential for proper cellular and hormonal function, but they also provide a concentrated source of energy in your diet that does not cause a surge in blood sugar or insulin, which means they help you lose excess pounds and maintain a healthy weight.

Saturated fats from animal and vegetable sources provide you with a number of important health benefits and help in the proper functioning of your:

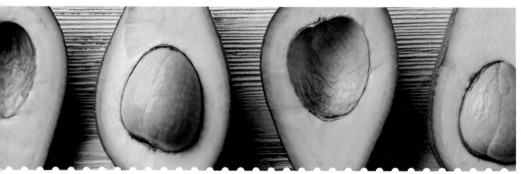

- Immune system
- Liver
- Cell membranes
- Bones
- Heart
- Hormones
- Lungs
- Genetic regulation

They also promote satiety, reducing your hunger pangs so you avoid binge eating and unhealthy food cravings. By following a high-fat, low-carb diet, you will be able to optimize your weight and avoid virtually all chronic degenerative diseases.

Fortunately, the low-fat recommendation, which flourished as a result of flawed science linking heart disease with saturated fat and the suppression of research showing sugar was to blame, is finally, albeit slowly, starting to lose its strong hold.

While still not ideal, the federal government's 2015–2020 Dietary Guidelines for Americans do recognize that reducing *total* fat intake has no bearing on obesity or heart disease risk.[4] Instead, the guidelines rightfully warn that sugar and refined grains are the primary culprits.

Unfortunately, the guidelines fall far short by still suggesting a 10 percent limit on saturated fats and recommending the use of skim milk and low-fat dairy products over full-fat versions, which I believe is a serious mistake. Low-fat recommendations are likely to do more harm than good across the board, but it may be particularly counterproductive for weight loss. In fact, mounting evidence clearly

shows that a high-fat, low-net-carb diet can be exceptionally effective for weight loss.

The key is to avoid processed foods, sugars, and grains as much as possible, and to make sure you're eating the right kind of fats, as all are not created equal. (I'll go more into the specific types of fats and other foods to eat more of in the next chapter.)

THE DANGER OF REPLACING SUGAR WITH DIET SODA AND ARTIFICIAL SWEETENERS

One of the most important steps you can take in recovering and maintaining your health is to drink clear, pure water. Drinking any type of soda can massively disrupt your ability to achieve health.

Considering the many health risks associated with obesity, the issue of whether artificially sweetened foods and beverages are a weight loss aid or hindrance is an important one. Many have fallen for industry claims suggesting that no- or low-calorie "diet" foods will help you lose weight and allow you to indulge in the sweeter side of life without harmful effects, but studies have repeatedly blown massive holes in these claims. Research has shown that artificial sweeteners produce a variety of metabolic dysfunctions that promote fat storage and weight gain, and many studies have directly associated artificial sweeteners with an increased risk of obesity, diabetes, and metabolic syndrome.[5]

Other mechanisms of harm have also been revealed. In recent years, we've learned that gut microbes play a significant role in human health. Certain gut microbes have been linked to obesity, for example, and research published in 2014 shows that artificial sweeteners raise your risk of obesity and diabetes by disrupting your intestinal microflora.[6]

The evidence suggests that artificial sweeteners have likely played a role in actually *worsening* the obesity and diabetes epidemics since their emergence in our food supply. And considering their many routes of harm, including disrupting your gut flora, I strongly recommend avoiding artificial sweeteners and reading food labels to make sure you're not inadvertently consuming them. They're added to some 6,000 different beverages, snacks, and food products, so there's no telling where they might be hiding.

If your favorite way to cut calories is to reach for a diet soda, know this: Research has confirmed again and again that diet soda tends to promote weight gain rather than prevent it. In a 2015 study, diet soda consumption was linked to increased belly fat in Americans over the age of 65.[7] An increase in belly fat is worse than simply gaining a few pounds: abdominal fat (visceral fat) is associated with an increased risk for diseases such as heart disease, diabetes, and cancer, to name just a few; in fact, your waist-to-hip ratio is one potent indicator of your level of risk for these and other chronic health problems.

In the 2015 study, people aged 65 and over were followed for an average of nine years, and while the research was observational and did not attempt to prove causation, the authors observed the following dose-response relationship between diet soda consumption and waist circumference:

- People who never drank diet soda increased their waist circumference by an average of 0.8 inches during the nine-year observation period.

- Occasional diet soda drinkers added an average of 1.83 inches to their waistline in that time period.

- Daily diet soda drinkers gained an average of nearly 3.2 inches—quadruple the gain of those who abstained from diet soda altogether.

This held true even when other factors such as exercise, diabetes, and smoking were taken into account. This isn't the first time diet soda has been linked to expanding waistlines. One 2011 study, in which soda drinkers were followed for nearly 10 years, found that those who drank diet soda had a 70 percent greater increase in waist size compared with those who did not drink it. And those who drank two or more diet sodas a day had a 500 percent greater increase in waist size.[8] And according to earlier research, drinking just one diet soda a day may raise the risk of obesity by 65 percent.

I hope this information will inspire you to break your diet soda habit, but don't expect it to be easy, as artificial sweeteners can be very addictive. Because no calories accompany the sweet flavor, your body receives no satisfaction on a cellular level when you consume artificial sweeteners, so your brain actually craves more. If you have trouble quitting diet soda or other artificially sweetened products, I suggest trying the Emotional Freedom Technique, which I cover in depth on my website at eft.mercola.com.

THE PATH TO WEIGHT LOSS

For decades now, you've been hearing that the undisputed formula for losing weight is to eat less—particularly less saturated fat—and exercise more. The cruel paradox is that you simply can't out-exercise your mouth, especially if you are eating low-fat and high-carb foods.

Remember, when you eat excessive high-net-carb foods, your pancreas releases insulin. Since excessive insulin cues your body to store calories as fat, high insulin prevents fat from being released. Furthermore, no amount of exercise can compensate for this. This is why it can seem nearly impossible to lose weight when you're eating processed foods filled with refined carbs and high-fructose corn syrup, and why cutting carbs is so critical when you're trying to lose weight.

So by following these flawed recommendations to eat less, especially less fat, and exercise more, we have inadvertently been doing the exact thing that causes weight gain.

The way out of this conundrum is simple and clear: get your body to burn fat as your primary fuel, as described in *Fat for Fuel*.

There are a few different reasons for this. First, as you start to burn fat for fuel, you free yourself from powerful cravings that may have made losing weight so challenging in the past. So not only do you lose weight, but it starts to feel downright effortless.

Making the transition to burning fat for fuel also releases a few pounds of water weight. When you are running on glucose, your body keeps some reserve glycogen (the stored form of glucose) safely tucked away in your skeletal muscle and your liver. When you stop eating non-fiber carbs, your body will use up these reserves before it starts burning fat. Each gram of glycogen is stored with three to four grams of water, and when the glycogen is burned that water is released, typically very soon after you begin restricting your carb intake.

After the initial quick water-weight loss that comes when you deplete your glycogen stores, your weight will trend downward until you reach your ideal weight.

When it comes to losing weight, a calorie *isn't* a calorie isn't a calorie. Changing the types of calories and the timing of when you eat them can help you heal insulin resistance and stop storing fat so you can start burning it. And you can do it without feeling deprived the way so many other diets make you feel.

5

OPTIMIZE YOUR NUTRITION

To protect your health, I recommend spending at least 90 percent of your food budget on whole foods and only 10 percent or less on processed foods. Unfortunately, most Americans currently do the opposite, which is in large part why so many struggle with junk food cravings. Remember, virtually *all* processed foods are to some degree designed to have a high "craveability" factor, and it's really difficult to find products that do not contain high amounts of addictive sugar and carbs. It's a self-perpetuating loop: as long as you are in carb-burning mode, you will strongly crave processed foods, and eating large amounts of processed foods will keep you in carb-burning mode.

The way off this merry-go-round is to replace the processed foods you eat with real foods, i.e., high-quality whole foods. Doing so will naturally leave less room on your plate for less-healthy choices. Also, by making those whole foods follow the high-fat, low-net-carb, adequate-protein ratios that I outline in this chapter, you will nudge your body to start burning fat as its primary source of fuel. And once that happens, your cravings for processed foods will dramatically diminish, if not vanish altogether.

I've outlined in this chapter the foods to avoid and the foods to celebrate in order to break the cycle of carb-burning and cravings. I know it may seem daunting at first, but I promise you that once you make the metabolic switch and experience what it feels like to be supported by the foods you eat instead of sickened, it won't feel like a sacrifice in the least—it will feel like a huge gain, and one that you were entirely responsible for creating.

FOODS TO AVOID

1. Sugar

Sweet, *tasty*, and *satisfying*—these are the words people often use to describe sugar. I, on the other hand, think of sugar as the exact opposite: *addictive*, *dangerous*, and *deadly*. Of all the foods capable of inflicting harm on your body, sugar is one of the most detrimental, which is why I'm mentioning it first here.

When I talk about sugar, I'm including *all* sugars, including honey, agave, table sugar, high-fructose corn syrup (HFCS), and the natural fructose found in fresh-pressed fruit juice and whole fruits. Many people are simply unaware of just how much sugar they're consuming, because it's not just candy, pastries, and soda that are loaded with added sugars—savory foods contain them as well. As do most, if not all, condiments, and even infant formula and baby food. Added sugar oftentimes hides under other, less familiar names, such as dextrose, maltose, galactose, and maltodextrin, for example. According to SugarScience.org, added sugars hide in 74 percent of processed foods under more than 60 different names.[1]

Adding insult to injury, sugar is also addictive. In fact, it's been shown to be more addictive than cocaine. Sugar hijacks the reward center in your brain, causing neurological changes identical to those seen in drug addicts and alcoholics.

For all these reasons, the U.S. Department of Agriculture (USDA) estimates that the average American consumed roughly 40 pounds of cane sugar and 25 pounds of high-fructose corn syrup in 2015 (the latest year for which numbers were available at the time of this writing).[2,3] These are numbers you simply must dramatically reduce if you want to lose weight and be—and stay—healthy.

Of all types of sugar, fructose takes the biggest toll on your health—even more than refined sugar does. Fructose is a sweetener usually derived from corn and is now the single largest calorie source for Americans. HFCS makes up 55 percent of the sweeteners used by food and beverage manufacturers today because it's cheaper and 20 percent sweeter than regular table sugar (sucrose). In fact, the number four source of calories in the United States today, across all age groups, is soda, which is sweetened with large amounts of HFCS. (The number one source of calories is grain-based desserts, which are also loaded with refined sugars and HFCS.)[4]

This is devastating for national health. Granted, *all* sugars contribute to weight gain to a certain degree, but highly refined and processed fructose, such as high-fructose corn syrup, wreaks the most biochemical havoc because it has the biggest negative impact on your leptin and insulin sensitivity, which results in metabolic syndrome. The bottom line is: fructose leads to increased visceral fat, insulin resistance, and metabolic syndrome—not to mention the long list of chronic diseases resulting from that.[5]

Fructose is more dangerous than glucose because every cell in your body utilizes glucose. Therefore, much of it is burned up immediately after you consume it. By contrast, cells don't use fructose for energy, so 100 percent of the fructose you eat is metabolized in your liver. When you eat 120 calories of glucose, less than one calorie is stored as fat; however, 120 calories of fructose results in 40 calories being stored as fat. On top of that, the metabolism of fructose by your liver creates a long list of waste products and toxins, including a large amount of uric acid, which drives

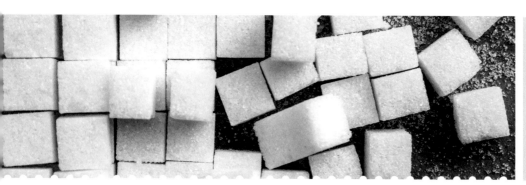

up blood pressure and causes gout. In short, fructose overconsumption damages your pancreas, liver, and brain much like alcohol does.

I hope these facts will help inspire you to break your sugar habit. Remember, when you have made the transition to burning fat, your cravings for sweets and processed foods will greatly lessen, if not disappear altogether, so it is doable.

2. Artificial sweeteners

As I discussed in the previous section on weight, artificial sweeteners actually contribute to weight gain, particularly a gain of dangerous visceral fat, and wipe out your populations of friendly gut bacteria. Of artificial sweeteners, aspartame is one of the worst.

Aspartame is the compound that goes by the brand names NutraSweet, Equal, Spoonful, and Equal-Measure. While it's one of the most commonly used artificial sweeteners in the world, it's also one of the most dangerous food additives, if not *the* most dangerous, on the market today.

Beyond its ties to obesity, when aspartame is in liquid form, it breaks down into methyl alcohol, or methanol, which is then converted into formaldehyde, which likely explains why aspartame accounts for over 75 percent of the adverse reactions to food additives reported to the FDA.

If you're looking for a way to sweeten your food that doesn't compromise your health, try stevia extract. It is derived from a South American plant of the same name and is very sweet—meaning that a little goes a long way. Another healthy sweetener is Lo han kuo, a Chinese fruit that is about 200 times sweeter than sugar. It is more expensive and harder to find than stevia. Erythritol and xylitol are two

sugar alcohols that have a much lower impact on blood sugar than traditional sugar and don't appear to have a detrimental effect on the microbiome. Just limit your use of these two so you don't become dependent on them. You can absolutely retrain your palate to not crave sweet foods, but not if you're adding an alternative sweetener to everything you eat.

3. Refined vegetable oils

Yes, you want to eat a high-fat diet in order to nudge your body into the fat-burning zone. But all fats are *not* created equal. The fats to avoid at all costs are processed vegetable oils, including corn, soy, safflower, sunflower, and canola oils. These vegetable oils consist of omega-6 fats, particularly linoleic acid. Omega-6 fats occur naturally in whole foods such as seeds and nuts and are essential nutrients that your body can't make, which is why they are called essential fatty acids (EFAs). While omega-6 fats in their natural, unrefined state are a vital part of a healthy diet, they need to make up only a relatively small percentage of your diet. You see, essential fats have double bonds that are highly susceptible to oxidative damage. So when you consume them, you are essentially rolling out the welcome mat for a free radical army that inflicts damage to your tissues, genes, and cell membranes. In other words, vegetable oils are highly inflammatory.

It is primarily for this reason that I believe the widespread consumption of refined vegetable oil is largely responsible for the epidemic of chronic disease that began in the 20th century, including heart disease, cancer, diabetes, and neurodegenerative diseases. There are other reasons I think this is so:

- **Omega-6:3 ratio.** There are two types of essential fats: omega-3s and omega-6s. The ratio of these fats in your body has profound signaling influences over a wide variety of metabolic processes. You should restrict your omega-6 intake to less than five times your intake of omega-3, or better yet, less than twice as much. That would be an omega-6:3 ratio of somewhere between 5:1 and 1:1—a ratio that reflects the diet of our ancestors, before the advent of refined vegetable oils. Because industrially processed omega-6 vegetable oils are cheap and widely used in processed foods, the average American now consumes 20 to 50 times more omega-6 oils than omega-3 oils, a ratio of 20:1 to 50:1.

- **Heating of oils.** As we've discussed, in their refined state omega-6 fats are highly unstable and susceptible to oxidative damage. Industrial refining further degrades their structure—first by heating them to high temperatures that alter their makeup; then by extracting them through toxic solvents, such as hexane, that then contaminate the oil; and then by further stripping them of any vital nutrients through steam distillation. Finally, cooking with these oils, especially at high heat, causes even more damage and creates a wide variety of toxic molecules.

- **Toxic herbicides.** The majority of the seeds used to make vegetable oil are now genetically modified—particularly corn, soy, and canola—meaning they are also now loaded with highly toxic chemical residues of the herbicide glyphosate (Roundup). This is because many GMO crops have been modified to be resistant to glyphosate—so farmers douse these plants with the herbicide knowing that the crops won't be killed; only the weeds will. While this practice may be good for the farm's bottom line, it's terrible for public health, as glyphosate has been demonstrated to have very serious detrimental impacts on cellular and microbiome health.

Sadly, these are the very fats that we have been advised to consume ever more of for several decades now—and are still counseled to use up until this very day.

4. Milk and yogurt

Today, most milk is produced in large concentrated animal feeding operations (CAFOs), where the animals don't receive sunlight, are fed genetically modified grains and soy products, and stand in one another's excrement. To ward off infection from these conditions, the animals are given antibiotics. They are also given steroids to boost their milk production. The milk must then be pasteurized in order to be safe for consumption. Unfortunately, the process of pasteurization kills most of the healthy enzymes and nutrients.

On top of this, most of the milk you'll find in the refrigerator case at your local grocery store has the butterfat purposefully removed to produce skim milk. Without butterfat your body can't absorb the fat-soluble vitamins that occur naturally in milk.

Truth be told, even whole milk isn't a great choice when you're trying to make the switch to burning fat, as it contains the dairy sugar lactose, which can worsen insulin and leptin resistance. (High-fat cheese, butter, cream, and ghee, on the other hand, can be healthful choices, particularly if they come from organically raised, grass-fed cows.)

Another type of dairy that is particularly problematic is most commercial yogurt, which is more akin to a sugary dessert than to a health food. Besides added sugar, typically in the form of high-fructose corn syrup, most commercial yogurts also contain artificial colors, flavors, and additives, all of which can harm beneficial microbes while nourishing disease-causing microorganisms in your gut. To top it off, much of the yogurt that is commercially available is low-fat and made from milk taken from conventionally raised CAFO cows, meaning it contains the antibiotics and hormones given to the cows.

While you do want to eat foods that contain probiotics—which I'll cover more in just a moment—conventional yogurts contain only small amounts of probiotics. In fact, a 2014 report from the Cornucopia Institute that evaluated commercially available yogurts found that the levels of probiotics they contained had little to do with what was promised on the labels.[6]

5. Unfermented soy

Despite what conventional health experts and health enthusiasts say, soy—particularly nonorganic, unfermented soy—is *not* good for you. In fact, it can weaken your immune system and lead to impaired thyroid function. Unfermented soy also contains phytoestrogens (or isoflavones) that are found to have adverse effects on human tissues and may lead to an increased risk of cancer.

Furthermore, 94 percent of soybeans grown in the United States are genetically modified, which can expose you to damaging herbicides like glyphosate.[7] This is associated with a host of negative effects and has been deemed a probable carcinogen that can cause non-Hodgkin's lymphoma and lung cancer in humans.

Avoiding unfermented soy products will also help you improve your omega-6:3 ratio, as soybean oil consists of omega-6 oils. Additionally, soybean and soy-based foods actually promote kidney stones in people prone to them, mainly because of their high levels of oxalates, which bind to calcium in your kidneys to form kidney stones.

6. Beans and legumes

Beans can provide you with good (but not complete) proteins. However, they are complex carbohydrates that can contribute to raising your insulin levels. They also contain a natural anti-nutrient called lectin, which I discussed in the Introduction.

Lectins (not to be confused with lecithin, which is a phospholipid) are carbohydrate-binding proteins, known as glycoproteins, that are widespread in the plant kingdom. An estimated 30 percent of fresh foods contain lectins.[8]

Lectins get their name from the Latin word *legere*, from which the word *select* derives—and that is exactly what they do: they select (attach to) specific biological structures that allow them to do harm, as part of the plant's self-defense mechanism. It's nature's ingenious way of keeping natural enemies like fungi and insects at bay. Unfortunately, some of these glycoproteins may also cause trouble in humans.

One major concern is that most lectins are inflammatory, meaning they trigger inflammation. They are also immunotoxic (capable of stimulating a hyperimmune response), neurotoxic, and cytotoxic, meaning they're toxic to cells and may induce apoptosis (cell death). Certain lectins may also increase your blood viscosity by binding to your red blood cells. Some lectins may even interfere with gene expression and disrupt endocrine function. Lectins also promote leptin resistance, thereby increasing your risk of obesity. All of these factors can predispose you to disease.

Beans not only contain lectins that can cause problems for many people, but also have the added drawback of being high in net carbs. They are therefore best avoided in the initial transitional stages of a ketogenic diet. Once you've fully made the transition to fat-burning, beans (and other net carbs such as grains) can be reincorporated, especially during your "feasting" days: Once your body is burning fat for fuel, you then begin cycling in and out of ketosis. As a general rule, I recommend increasing your net carbs and protein one or two days a week—days on which you can go as high as 100 grams or more of net carbs—and then cycling back into ketosis on the remaining five or six days. During these high-carb days, beans are acceptable if you like and can tolerate them, but they must be cooked in a modern, high-quality pressure cooker such as an Instant Pot to reduce lectins.

7. Grains

Many people rely on grains for a large portion of their calories, and whole grains have been heralded as a health food by mainstream media and health experts. Still, even whole grains can raise your insulin and leptin levels. Grains have been linked to a host of health conditions, such as gluten sensitivity, autoimmune diseases, Alzheimer's disease, and autism. Grains may also worsen symptoms such as brain fog, skin rashes, fatigue, joint pain, and allergies. Digestive ailments (bloating, gas, and abdominal cramps) have also been linked to grain consumption. And if you are harboring pathogenic microbes, the fiber in grains can serve as "food" for them, worsening your ailments. In addition, most grains are loaded with toxins, such as lectin, which is also found in beans.

If the thought of life without staples such as bread, pasta, and rice is making you nervous, know that there are grain-free substitutes for these popular foods—see pages 154, 224, and 231 for ideas to get you started.

(The one grain that is virtually toxin-free is white rice, which has far fewer toxins than brown rice. After you're fat-adapted, you may decide to eat it on your feast days.)

8. Trans fats

Six decades ago, the food industry began replacing many saturated fats (such as lard) with more shelf-stable trans fats (such as partially hydrogenated soybean oil)—and the processed food movement was born.

Americans' health has plummeted ever since, and millions have been prematurely killed by this mistake. Making matters worse, genetically engineered soy oil, which is a major source of trans fat, can oxidize inside your body, thereby causing damage to both your heart and your brain.

In 2007, when New York City severely limited the amount of trans fat allowed to be served at restaurants, it offered a unique opportunity for researchers to study the effects on residents in the counties where the ban was in effect and compare rates of hospital admissions for heart attack and stroke in those counties before and after the restriction to rates of hospital admissions for heart attack and stroke in other New York State counties where there were no restrictions on trans fats.[9] Three or more years after the restrictions were imposed on specific counties, researchers found a 6.2 percent reduction in hospital admissions for heart attacks and stroke in those counties compared with areas of the state where the restrictions on trans fat were not imposed.

The primary sources of trans fat in processed food are often indicated as "partially hydrogenated" palm, cottonseed, soybean, vegetable, and canola oils. Unfortunately, they hide in many processed foods you may have at home. Flaky crusts for your pies are often made with vegetable shortening loaded with partially hydrogenated oil. Artificial creamers, frozen dairy desserts, and cake icing are just a couple of places where partially hydrogenated oils hide, providing the "creaminess" in thoroughly processed foods.

The public is now largely aware of the risk of trans fats, and many manufacturers have stopped relying on trans fats as their main source of fat. But it is still fairly easy to eat well over 1 gram of trans fat each day. FDA labeling rules allow manufacturers to list the amount of trans fat as 0 percent if there is less than 0.5 grams per serving in the product.[10] While you may think that sounds reasonable, manufacturers are able to exploit this rule by changing portion sizes. By reducing the portion size, they reduce the amount of trans fat found in each serving, thus fulfilling FDA rules for the "zero trans fat" label. In fact, they may even announce on the label that the product does not have trans fat. So make it a habit to read the fine print on any processed foods you purchase. If the serving size is ridiculously small, this is a tip-off you may be getting trans fat after all.

9. Potato chips and french fries

Potatoes are the most consumed vegetable in America. This is a problem for three reasons: These starchy vegetables contain plenty of simple sugars that are rapidly converted to glucose, which raises insulin levels and can contribute to insulin resistance. In addition, conventionally grown potatoes are among the highest in pesticide contents of any fruit or vegetable. In fact, the USDA reports that the amount of pesticides used on one acre of potato plants has increased exponentially, from 6.6 pounds in 1960 to 44 pounds in 1999 to nearly 50 pounds in 2008.[11] And finally, when potatoes are cooked at high heat—as when they are turned into potato chips or French fries—a potentially neurotoxic chemical called acrylamide is created.

Acrylamide is the by-product of a chemical reaction between sugars and the amino acid asparagine, which occurs at high temperatures. While the chemical can form in many foods cooked or processed at temperatures above 250 degrees F (120 degrees C), carbohydrate-rich foods are by far the most vulnerable.

In November 2013, the FDA issued a consumer update advising people to reduce consumption of foods in which acrylamide is plentiful, noting this toxic by-product is found in 40 percent of calories consumed by the average American.[12]

Potato chips and french fries are some of the worst acrylamide offenders. Not only do you have acrylamide to contend with, but unless they are fried in coconut oil or lard, you're also getting a hefty dose of harmful vegetable oil.

10. Conventionally raised meat, poultry, and eggs

In concentrated animal feeding operations (CAFOs), with animals packed into tight quarters, fed unnatural diets, and living in filth, disease flourishes. Low doses of antibiotics are added to feed as a matter of course, not only to stave off infectious diseases but also because they cause the animals to grow faster on less food. In fact, 80 percent of the antibiotics used in the United States are used by industrial agriculture for purposes of growth promotion and prevention of diseases that would otherwise make CAFOs unviable. The problem is, while the antibiotics may kill most of the bacteria in the animals, the remaining, resistant bacteria are allowed to survive and multiply.

In addition, animals raised in CAFOs are typically fed grains, such as corn or soybeans, that tend to be genetically modified and doused in pesticides. Also, grains aren't the animals' natural foods, so they don't get all the nutrients they need. As a result, meat and eggs from these conventionally raised animals aren't as nutritious as their organic, grass-fed counterparts (see pages 44–45 for more information).

FOODS TO CELEBRATE

1. Healthy saturated fats

Saturated fats from animal and vegetable sources are an important component of the Fat for Fuel program, as they provide you with a number of important health benefits and help in the proper functioning of your immune system, cell membranes, heart, lungs, liver, bones, hormones, and genetic regulation. Saturated fats also promote satiety, reducing your hunger pangs so you avoid binge eating and unhealthy food cravings.

So what is good fat, and how can you distinguish it from unhealthy forms? In general, full-fat, raw (i.e., unpasteurized), grass-fed butter, cheese, and ghee; olives and authentic olive oil; coconut oil; raw nuts such as macadamias and pecans; organic, pastured eggs; avocados; grass-fed meats; MCT oil; pastured chicken fat (schmaltz), lard, and tallow; and raw cacao are all great sources of healthy fats.

One of my favorite sources of healthy fats are avocados, which are low in fructose and rich in healthy monounsaturated fat, making them an ideal cornerstone of a fat-burning diet. They provide close to 20 essential health-boosting nutrients, including vitamin E, B vitamins, and folic acid. They are also excellent sources of fiber and potassium. I personally eat as many as three avocados a day—they are satiating and delicious. Research has found that avocados can be beneficial for weight loss and appear to help regulate blood sugar and fight cancer.[13,14] Because of their thick skin, they are resistant to pesticide contamination, meaning you don't necessarily need to spend more to buy organic.

The only drawback to avocados is that they are expensive. A way to make them more budget-friendly is to purchase them in bulk when they're on sale—choose the avocados that are entirely green and rock-hard, then store them in the fridge, where they will last up to three weeks. Simply take them out of the refrigerator two or three days before you want to eat them.

2. Fiber

There are two types of fiber, soluble and insoluble. Insoluble fiber is bulkier and can help prevent constipation. Further, it has no impact on your caloric intake, blood sugar, or insulin levels.[15] Soluble fiber dissolves and forms a gel-like substance that helps food move smoothly through your system, making you feel full. Soluble fiber is fermented by bacteria into short-chain fatty acids (SCFAs), which do not increase blood glucose and may even help reduce blood sugar levels.[16]

Many whole foods, especially fruits and vegetables, naturally contain both soluble and insoluble fiber. This is ideal, as both help feed the microorganisms living in your gut. To meet your daily fiber requirements, you'll want to eat plenty of non-starchy, organic vegetables, nuts, and seeds.

I am a major fan of fiber, especially soluble fibers like psyllium, as they not only serve as a prebiotic for your microbiome but are also metabolized to short-chain fatty acids like butyrate, propionic acid, and acetate, which nourish your colonic cells. They are also converted to ketones that nourish your tissues.

Dietary guidelines call for 20 to 30 grams of fiber per day, but I believe an ideal amount for most adults is likely much higher, perhaps twice as much. I personally consume nearly 100 grams of fiber a day, including about 2 tablespoons of organic psyllium three times a day, which provides about 25 grams of soluble fiber. The other 75 percent of my fiber comes primarily from vegetables and seeds.

3. Low-net-carb vegetables

As a general rule, vegetables are a nutritional cornerstone. Most vegetables are very low in calories and net carbs while high in healthy fiber and the valuable vitamins and minerals your body needs for optimal health. Vegetables also contain an array of antioxidants and other disease-fighting compounds that are very difficult to get anywhere else. Plant chemicals called phytochemicals help reduce inflammation and eliminate carcinogens, while others regulate the rate at which your cells reproduce, remove old cells, and maintain DNA. The fiber content of vegetables also promotes optimal gut health in general by nourishing beneficial gut bacteria.

You can eat as many of these vegetables, which are high in fiber and low in carbohydrate content, as you like:

- Asparagus
- Avocados
- Broccoli
- Brussels sprouts
- Cabbage

- Cauliflower
- Celery
- Kale
- Mushrooms
- Salad greens
- Sauté greens
- Spinach

After you have successfully made the transition to burning fat, you can add back limited amounts of these vegetables:

- Garlic
- Onions
- Parsnips
- Peppers
- Rutabaga
- Tomatoes
- Winter squash (very limited amounts)

4. Fermented foods

A great way to eat more vegetables, particularly in the winter months when fewer fresh vegetables are available, is to ferment them.

Fermented foods have been part of the human diet since ancient times. They are potent chelators, or detoxifiers, and very rich sources of probiotics. In fact, eating fermented foods can provide more probiotics than taking a supplement can. Eating fermented vegetables, such as sauerkraut or kimchi, combines the high fiber of vegetables with the probiotics of fermented foods.

Start by adding as little as one teaspoon of fermented vegetables with every meal. It may seem like a small amount, but it will have a dramatically beneficial impact on your health. You can increase this amount gradually over a few weeks or months, aiming for one-quarter to one-half cup of fermented vegetables with every meal. Do not be tempted to start off with a large amount, though, as too large a portion may provoke a healing crisis. This occurs when the good bacteria kill off pathogens in your gut, which then release potent toxins. Adjust your portions gradually and listen to your body.

Fermented vegetables offer a host of benefits, but remember that variety is important, in order to inoculate your gut with a mix of different species of microorganisms. So aside from cultured vegetables, try these other fermented foods:

- Chutneys
- Fish, such as fermented mackerel and Swedish gravlax
- Natto
- Tempeh

In my view, optimizing your gut health is a foundational step if you are seeking to achieve good overall health. Addressing your gut flora is also important for most health conditions, be they acute or chronic. While you could certainly benefit from a high-quality probiotic supplement, eating fermented foods is, I believe, a more effective and far less expensive option.

5. Nuts

Macadamia nuts have the highest fat and lowest protein and carbohydrate content of any nut. One ounce of macadamia nuts has only four grams of carbs, but more than half of those are nondigestible fiber, leaving an ultra-low two grams of sugar per ounce of nuts. They also contain high amounts of vitamin B1, magnesium, and manganese. Just one serving of macadamia nuts offers 58 percent of what you need in manganese and 23 percent of the recommended daily value of thiamin.

Moreover, about 60 percent of the fatty acid in macadamias is the monounsaturated fat oleic acid, which is an omega-9. This is about the level found in olives, which are well known for their health benefits.

Macadamia nuts make a great snack. They are easily portable, don't require refrigeration (so you can keep them in your glove compartment or desk drawer), and can help keep your fat intake up—and your hunger down. They also happen to be my favorite nut.

Pecans are a close second to macadamia nuts on the fat and protein scale, and they also contain anti-inflammatory magnesium, heart-healthy oleic acid, phenolic antioxidants, and immune-boosting manganese. Pecans contain more than 19 vitamins and minerals, and research has shown they may help lower low-density lipoprotein (LDL), or the "bad" type of cholesterol, and promote healthy arteries. They are also in the top 15 foods identified by the USDA as high in antioxidants. Like macadamia nuts, pecans are not only a healthy snack but a convenient one, due to their portability.

6. Seeds

Seeds contain everything a plant needs to grow, and consequently, they are among the most nutrient-dense foods you can find. They are great sources of protein, fiber, minerals, vitamins, antioxidants, and omega-3 fats (in the case of flax and chia seeds), all rolled up into one tiny package. Many seeds also contain compounds known as lignans, which are substances that can help promote hormone balance in the body.

One caveat with seeds is that most are loaded with lectins and should be avoided unless they are sprouted or soaked overnight, as this will radically reduce the lectins. Another concern is that seeds are natural

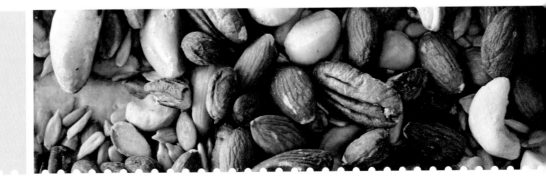

sources of omega-6 fats; you'll want to limit your intake of seeds to a moderate amount so that you don't throw off your omega-3/omega-6 ratios. Like nuts, seeds travel well, and they make a great addition to smoothies, salads, and soups. They are also good in a homemade trail mix with macadamias and/or pecans. The following are the seeds I eat and recommend you consider for yourself. Eat up to three tablespoons of a combination of seeds daily:

- Black cumin
- Black sesame
- Chia seeds (high in lectins, though, so avoid these if you are autoimmune-challenged, or soak them before using)
- Flax seeds, ground
- Psyllium seed husks
- Pumpkin seeds
- Sunflower seeds

7. Animal-based omega-3 fats

Omega-3 fats are essential for optimal brain health. However, few people get enough through diet and instead overload on polyunsaturated omega-6 fats.

One of the easiest ways to maintain your omega-6:3 ratio is to regularly eat healthy fish like Alaskan salmon, sardines, and anchovies. They are high in omega-3s and generally safe from contamination, since they are not allowed to be farmed and therefore are always wild-caught. What's more, sockeye salmon has a short life cycle, which reduces its

risk of accumulating high amounts of mercury and other toxins.

When purchasing salmon, make sure you are buying "Alaskan salmon" or "wild Alaskan salmon" or "sockeye salmon." Canned varieties labeled "Alaskan salmon" are also recommended and are an inexpensive alternative to fillets.

Also look for the Marine Stewardship Council (MSC) certification. This assures that every component of the manufacturing process, from harvesting the raw materials to manufacturing and packaging, has been scrutinized by a third party.

Another factor to consider when purchasing salmon is evaluating how it looks. The flesh of wild sockeye salmon is bright red, courtesy of its natural astaxanthin content. It's also very lean, so the fat marks, those white stripes you see in the meat, are very thin. If the fish is pale pink with wide fat marks, the salmon was farmed. Avoid salmon labeled "Atlantic salmon" because typically this comes from fish farms.

8. Organic, pastured eggs

Eggs are one of the all-around most nutritious forms of food on the planet. They contain high-quality proteins, fats, vitamins, and minerals. The yolks are rich in lutein and zeaxanthin, a class of plant pigments (they give the yolks their orange and yellow hues) known as xanthophylls that offer powerful prevention against age-related macular degeneration, which is the most common cause of blindness. Also present are naturally occurring B12, choline, and amino acids such as tryptophan and tyrosine, which have potent antioxidant properties that help prevent cardiovascular disease and cancer.

Free-range, or pastured, organic eggs are far superior when it comes to nutrient content. An egg is considered organic if the laying chicken has been fed only organic food, which means it has not accumulated high levels of pesticides from the grains (mostly GM corn) typically fed to chickens.

Cooking destroys many of the nutrients, so ideally, you'll want to consume your eggs lightly cooked or raw in a healthy, fat-rich homemade treat affectionately known as a "fat bomb" (see recipe on page 258) or in a smoothie, but only if they're pastured organic. Conventionally raised eggs are far more likely to be contaminated with disease-causing bacteria such as salmonella and should be avoided.

9. Sprouts

One of the most vital, health-promoting foods you can eat are sprouted seeds—my favorites are sunflower, broccoli, and pea sprouts. These baby plants contain as much as 30 times the nutritional density of typical vegetables. As a result, you need to eat far less of them to get the same benefit.

You can even grow your own, making them extremely cost-effective as well as life-affirming; they can grow on a sunny windowsill in just a few days, even in the middle of winter. Eating sprouts makes it much easier to eat your daily allotment of vegetables—you can consume them as a salad, replacing the lettuce, or add them to your green juice. For detailed instructions on how to grow your own sprouts, visit Mercola.com and search for "How to Grow Your Own Food in Small Spaces."

10. Kale

Kale is a well-recognized "superfood." It is rich in healthy fiber and antioxidants, and it is one of the best sources of vitamin A, which promotes eye and skin health and may help strengthen your immune system, and vitamin K.

A 1-cup serving has almost as much vitamin C as an orange and as much calcium as a cup of milk. It's also an excellent source of lutein and zeaxanthin (which help protect against macular degeneration), indole-3-carbinol (thought to protect against colon cancer by aiding DNA repair), iron, and chlorophyll.

One serving of kale also contains 2 grams of protein, 121 milligrams (mg) of plant-based omega-3 fats, 92 mg of omega-6, and—like meat—all nine essential amino acids needed to form proteins in your body, plus nine non-essential ones. Studies suggest kale can help lower total cholesterol and LDL cholesterol while raising levels of high-density lipoprotein (HDL, or "good") cholesterol, thus lessening your risk for heart disease. Kale has also been shown to provide "comprehensive support" for detoxification by regulating the process at the genetic level.

11. Grass-fed beef

There's a lot of confusion about the term *grass-fed*. In many cases, it's an abused term like the word *natural*. Some producers of beef will misuse this term because the rules around it are still somewhat undefined. It's important to recognize that while the USDA 100% Organic label is good, it's not necessarily a guarantee that the meat has been fed grass its entire life. *Grass-fed* only means that cows started off eating grass—they may have been fed grain during the winters to supplement when grass wasn't abundant and/or during the last few months of their lives to fatten them up before slaughter. *Grass-finished* means the cows were fed only grass and whatever they could forage from the pasture for their entire lives. In my mind, a truly grass-fed, grass-finished product is superior to organic. There is a new certification called American Grass Fed Association. Look for this certification to confirm you are getting authentic grass-finished beef.

Some of the benefits of grass-fed and grass-finished beef include higher levels of conjugated linoleic acid (CLA) and other healthy fats; it's also free of antibiotics and other drugs used in CAFOs. With antibiotic-resistant disease being a major public health hazard, buying organic meats is an important consideration in more ways than one.

Unless labeled as grass-fed, virtually all the meat you buy in the grocery store is CAFO beef, and tests have revealed that nearly half of the meat sold in U.S. stores is contaminated with pathogenic bacteria—including antibiotic-resistant strains. Grass-fed beef is not associated with this high frequency of contamination, and the animals' living conditions have everything to do with this improved safety.

Nearly all calves are fed grass for a certain amount of time. This is one factor that allows less scrupulous producers to get away with calling their beef grass-fed. The key to a truly grass-fed product is actually the finishing. Optimal beef is both grass-fed and grass-finished. The only way to be sure that your meat has been grass-finished is to know the farms and the farmers that produce it. For this reason, the best place to buy meat is from local farms, a farmer's market, or a trusted online source that buys and ships directly from the producers.

12. Bone broth

Homemade bone broth is a nutritional powerhouse that can go a long way toward improving your diet and health. It also tastes great whether you sip it on its own or turn it into soup. Bone broth is made from simmering the bones of animals—such as chicken, cows, lamb, or fish—for at least six hours and as long as two days. When the bones are cooked this long, they release their minerals, vitamins, and other nutrients. These include calcium, magnesium, phosphorus, silicon, sulfur, collagen, glycine, glutamine, trace minerals, and compounds like chondroitin and glucosamine, which are sold as expensive supplements for arthritis and joint pain. Good old-fashioned bone broth fights inflammation, promotes healthy digestion, boosts immunity, and promotes strong bones, hair, and nails. Sipping it can also help rebalance electrolytes, making it an effective "sports drink."

THE IMPORTANCE OF NUTRITIONAL COMPOSITION

Focusing your diet on raw, whole, and ideally organic foods rather than processed fare is one of the easiest ways to sidestep dietary pitfalls like excess sugar/fructose, harmful trans fats, genetically modified organisms (GMOs), and harmful additives while getting plenty of healthy nutrients. The rest is a matter of tweaking the ratios of fat, net carbs, and protein to suit your individual situation.

In order to make the switch to burning fat for fuel—and to enjoy the benefits of weight optimization and disease prevention that this switch offers—you need to eat a diet that is high in healthy fats, adequate in protein, and low in net carbs.

Good Health Starts by Counting Net Carbs

The reason it's so important to limit your net carbs is that high-sugar foods will cause your blood sugar to rise, and glucose is an inherently "dirty" fuel that generates large amounts of inflammation-causing free radicals—far more than fat does when burned.

As I've said before, net carbs are defined as total carbs minus fiber. In order to convert to burning fat for fuel, you need to radically limit your intake of net carbs to 50 grams per day or less. In order to do this and still feel satisfied and full and get all the energy your body needs to function, you should replace the calories you would otherwise be consuming as carbs with healthy fats. Making this dietary switch will transition your body into primarily burning fat for fuel and will radically reduce your risk for most chronic diseases.

For the greatest success on this eating plan, make your primary source of net carbs organic vegetables (refer back to pages 41–42 for a list of suitable options), as they provide fiber and many vitamins and antioxidants and have a minimal impact on blood sugar levels.

Protein Is Important, but in the Right Amounts

Protein and its array of amino acids are the primary building blocks of your muscles, bones, enzymes, and many hormones. You simply cannot live without protein. But can you eat *too much* protein?

The answer is a resounding, definitive yes. There is an upper limit to how much protein your body can use to replenish and repair your muscles, and if you do not regularly stay within this limit, it will spell trouble for your health.

As I discussed on page 7, excessive protein intake stimulates the mTOR pathway, one of the most important signaling pathways in your body, which can in turn promote the growth of cancer cells. As long as you keep your protein intake at an adequate level to meet your body's needs without consuming an excess, the mTOR pathway is inhibited, which then reduces your risk of cancer growth.

So how much protein do you actually need each day? You likely need about one-half gram of protein per pound of lean body mass. This amounts to 30 to 70 grams, spread out throughout the day. If you're aggressively exercising or competing, or pregnant or lactating, your daily protein requirement may be 25 to 50 percent higher.

To calculate your lean body mass, subtract your percentage of body fat from 100. So if you have 20 percent body fat, then you have 80 percent lean body mass. Then multiply that percentage (in this case, 0.8) by your current weight to get your lean body mass in pounds. In this example, if you weigh 160 pounds, multiply that amount by 0.8 (80 percent), which leaves you with 128 pounds of lean body mass. Following the rule to consume one-half gram of protein per pound per day, you would need about 64 grams of protein per day.

Note that 64 grams of protein does not represent a large amount of food. It can be as little as two small hamburger patties or a six-ounce chicken breast. Check out this list as a simple guide on the grams of protein in foods:

Red meat, pork, poultry, and seafood average 6 to 9 grams of protein per ounce, meaning a 3-ounce serving will provide 18 to 27 grams of protein. I hope this will help you reconsider eating 9- or 12-ounce steaks!

One egg contains 6 to 8 grams of protein, so an omelet made from two eggs would give you 12 to 16 grams of protein. If you add cheese, you need to calculate that protein in as well (check the nutritional info on the label of your cheese).

Seeds and nuts contain, on average, 4 to 8 grams of protein per quarter cup.

Cooked beans average about 7 to 8 grams per half cup.

Once you are burning fat for fuel, it is wise to stimulate mTOR one to two times per week when you are strength training. This is best done with additional branched chained amino acids, especially leucine. One of the best ways to do this is with a high-quality grass-fed whey protein concentrate that is particularly high in leucine. In addition to carefully considering the amount of protein you eat, you need to consider its source. Be wary of meats sold in conventional markets, as they mostly come from CAFOs.

And finally, in addition to limiting the total amount of protein you eat each day, you also should be mindful of spreading that protein consumption out throughout the day, aiming to consume no more than 12 to 20 grams of protein in any given meal. This will help prevent any excess protein from being converted into glucose and help keep your blood sugar and insulin levels down.

Healthy Saturated Fat

For optimal health, you may need anywhere from 50 to 80 percent of your daily calories in the form of healthy fats. Remember, this means eating high-quality *saturated* fats and avoiding refined vegetable oils and trans fats as much as you possibly can. Refer back to page 40 for the list of healthy fats. The recipes included in this book are all formulated to help you reach this level of healthy fat intake, so pick two or three that appeal to your palate and start there. Apart from the recipes, coconut oil and avocados can be very efficient ways of upping your total intake of healthy fats—you can eat an avocado plain with a sprinkling of sea salt and a squeeze of lemon juice for a satisfying snack. Also, see the recipe for Chocolate Fat Bomb on page 258 for a delicious snack that delivers a hefty amount of high-quality fat in just a couple of bites.

THE IMPORTANCE OF LOGGING YOUR MEALS

Keeping a record of the food you eat is a powerful way to help you make better food choices. If you know you're going to need to write down that chocolate croissant, for example, that knowledge alone may be enough to steer you toward a healthier, lower-net-carb choice.

Beyond simple recording, tracking your food with a high-tech tool can help you determine the nutritional composition of your diet at a glance, without needing to do any complicated calculating on your own. If you're making the commitment to burn fat for fuel, an online nutrient tracker is the easiest, most efficient way to determine your net carb intake, and Cronometer is one of the best. It's also completely free.

Cronometer is far more than your typical calorie-counting diet app. This comprehensive website and app for your mobile device (so you can use it on the go) makes it easy to track the food you eat and, even more important, to see at a glance the nutritional makeup of that food. Not only will it tell you how much fat, protein, and carbohydrates you've eaten on any given day, both in total grams and percentages of your total calories, but it can track more than 40 micronutrients, with a focus on nutrition analysis. You can see if you're deriving sufficient fiber or omega-3s from the food you eat, for example, or if you should supplement to get your levels up. No other tool maintains such a detailed nutrition database or can analyze your data in such detail.

Another valuable benefit of using Cronometer is that you can plan your meals and enter the information before you actually eat. Additionally, the site offers discussion forums and a blog that cover a wide range of topics regarding your health journey, from the ketogenic diet to the importance of vitamin D to new applications.

I liked Cronometer so much that I worked with the developer for months to modify and optimize the program for the low-net-carb, adequate-protein, and high-fat diet that I espouse in *Fat for Fuel*. The Cronometer mobile app is available for iOS and Android and offers easy-to-use touch-screen optimization so that even when you're out and about, its streamlined data entry site is readily accessible.

Furthermore, by entering your personal health data and biomarkers, such as your glucose readings, you can also participate in an important research project that will analyze the data to assess the impact and effectiveness of this dietary intervention. This is the kind of research that really needs to be done in order to validate the effectiveness of this approach and turn our current disease epidemics around. All of your information is anonymous, of course, and you're under no obligation to enter any specific data.

To get started using Cronometer, create an account and log in. You'll be able to access helpful videos in the User Manual that show you how to use the service. From there, you can start logging your food and entering your biometrics. I think you will find it fascinating to see how the food you eat translates to nutrients consumed.

Needless to say, to get the most out of this analytic tool you need to *use it*. Ideally, use it daily, at least for a finite period of time (I suggest at least three months). It's important to understand that it's not something you'll have to do daily for the rest of your life; it's just a short-term intervention.

A tracker like Cronometer may be the key you need for optimizing your nutrition so you feel good and look good and are not always wondering what you're missing. It eliminates the guesswork, allowing you to get a truly accurate and detailed analysis of what you're eating. It will help change your relationship with food from one that's more emotional and subject to cravings to one that's based on an enlightened understanding of which foods truly fuel you and your health.

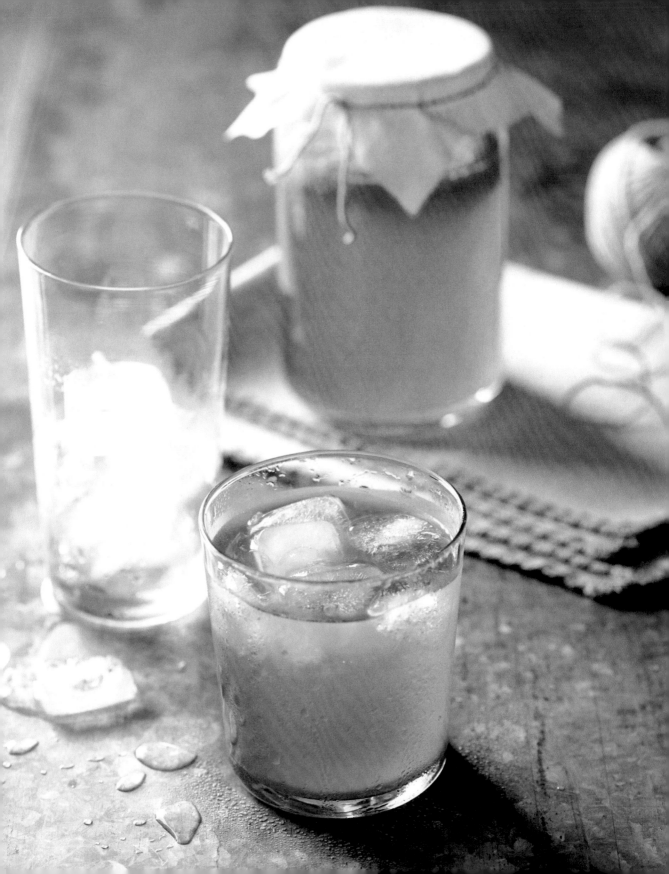

UPGRADE YOUR BEVERAGES

Making the transition to burning fat isn't just about eating the right foods and eating at the right time. It also requires drinking the right beverages. I doubt you will be surprised to learn that you'll need to completely wean yourself off soda, juice, and store-bought energy drinks. No matter how cleverly they are marketed, these beverages won't do your body any favors. They are typically loaded with sugar and/or artificial sweeteners and food dye. They may also contain excessive amounts of caffeine that can lead to dehydration, or worse.

What should you drink, then? I believe that no beverage can quench thirst and support health better than pure, filtered, or natural spring water. After all, water makes up 65 percent of your body and helps with blood circulation, metabolism, body temperature regulation, waste removal, and detoxification. Simply put, you need water to survive and thrive.

The best water you could possibly drink would come from a natural spring. Spring water molecules are structured in a slightly different way from your typical water, which is why it's also known as structured water or living water. Structured water is the water your body needs to function optimally, and your cells are mainly composed of it. If you happen to live near a natural spring or have the opportunity to visit one (go to FindaSpring.org for guidance), I encourage you to fill up. Store the water in glass jars so toxic chemicals and substances cannot get into it.

Although not everyone has access to a spring, you can still have your own supply of structured water by cooling water to about 39 degrees Fahrenheit (4 degrees Centigrade) or stirring the water with a spoon in a circular jar to make a vortex; this will help rearrange the water molecules and give them more structure.

If you don't have access to spring water, use filtered tap water. Make sure to buy a filter that is easy to use and effective and gives you value for your money. My personal recommendation is a reverse osmosis (RO) filter, which removes more impurities than other types of water filter systems.

TYPES OF WATER TO AVOID

There are three types of water you should try to avoid: fluoridated, distilled, and bottled. It is easier to say to avoid fluoridated water than to actually do it, since most municipal water supplies in the United States are treated with fluoride. I strongly oppose water fluoridation because fluoride has been linked to a host of problems including thyroid disorders, attention-deficit hyperactivity disorder, and learning and memory problems. Fluoride negatively impacts IQ levels too, and it has been labeled an endocrine disruptor. Reverse osmosis water filters can remove fluoride; look into installing one in your home, as it will provide a lot of benefit with little cost or inconvenience.

I recommend avoiding most distilled water because the distillation process increases the amount of toxic substances, especially disinfection by-products (DBPs). DBPs are 10,000 times more toxic than chlorine and are the worst toxins in water. Additionally, the distillation process causes the water to lose its structure. Distilled water is also both acidic and demineralized and can provoke leakage of contaminants into the water. Some of the equipment used to distill water is made of metal, so toxic substances like nickel may be added. If the distiller uses a plastic bottle, BPA and phthalates can leach into the water as well.

The plastics used for bottled water are actually an opportunity for dangerous chemicals like bisphenol A (BPA), bisphenol S (BPS), and phthalates. BPA and BPS are estrogen-mimicking chemicals linked to reproductive defects, learning and behavioral problems, immune dysfunction, and prostate and breast cancer.[1,2,3,4,5] Phthalates are endocrine disruptors linked to developmental and reproductive effects and reduced IQ in children.[6]

In addition, bottled water is an environmental nuisance because of the waste it produces and is economically impractical and deceiving. The National Resources Defense Council estimates bottled water costs as much as 10,000 times more per gallon than regular tap water, and that 25 percent of bottled water is nothing more than regular tap water that has undergone no additional filter treatments.[7]

HOW TO KNOW YOU'RE DRINKING ENOUGH

Regarding how much water to drink, let your thirst mechanism and the color and quantity of your urine be your guide. The thirst signal is the most important and kicks in when your body loses 1 to 2 percent of its total water content. The only caution about depending too much on thirst is that you'll only feel it when you're already a bit dehydrated, so be sure to monitor your urine color and quantity too.

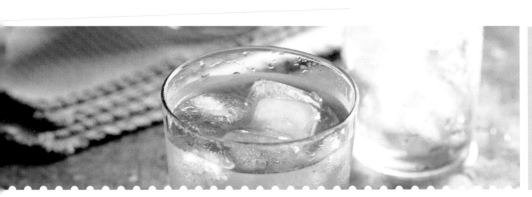

If your urine is pale yellow, you're likely drinking enough. Dark-colored urine means you may be dehydrated, leading your kidneys to retain fluids to maintain fluid-dependent bodily functions. Bright-colored urine, on the other hand, may be triggered by vitamin B2, found in most multivitamins. The frequency of your toilet trips is another factor. Ideally, you should urinate about seven to eight times a day. If you're not urinating enough or if hours go by between trips, it's probably time to drink more water.

 Sipping water throughout the day is preferable to drinking large amounts at one time, since your body is able to process only about one eight-ounce glass of water per hour. If you drink more, the water won't be used, and it'll be flushed down the drain, taking valuable electrolytes with it.

OTHER HEALTHY BEVERAGES

Vegetable juicing is a great way to reach your daily requirement of vegetables, and you get them in their raw form. When you drink freshly made green juice or a vegetable smoothie, it is almost like getting an intravenous infusion of vitamins, minerals, and enzymes—they go straight into your system without having to be broken down.

If you're new to juicing, start with mild-tasting veggies like celery. From there you can begin to add romaine lettuce, red leaf lettuce, fennel, spinach, parsley, and cilantro. When you start to include greens like collard greens, kale, dandelion greens, and mustard greens, you'll notice that they can taste quite bitter, so add just a few leaves at a time. For flavor and sweetness, you can add the following:

- **Limes and lemons.** Add one half to a whole lime or lemon for every quart of juice. You can juice the skins as well as the flesh.

- **Cranberries.** Limit them to about four ounces per pint of juice.

- **Fresh ginger.** This gives your juice a mildly spicy kick. Ginger has other health benefits as well, including lowering blood glucose.

Make sure that organic green vegetables, and not fruits, make up the bulk of your juice. Otherwise it will be high in calories and sugar. It can take time to get used to the strong flavor of green juice, but you can tweak it to fit your palate.

Coffee is another beverage that can have therapeutic benefits, as long as it's *high-quality* and *organic*. This is important, as nonorganic coffee is typically heavily sprayed with pesticides. The coffee plant, including its beans (which are actually seeds), contains a natural blend of polyphenol antioxidants—such as chlorogenic acids, bioflavonoids, vitamins, and minerals—that all provide impressive health-promoting benefits. The combination of these elements is so potent that it can actually moderate the harsher effects of naturally occurring caffeine in coffee.

Research has found that coffee may have a protective effect on your heart. A study of more than 25,000 people found that those who drank three to five cups of coffee daily were less likely to have calcium deposits in their coronary arteries than were those who drank either no coffee or more coffee daily.[8] Other studies found that coffee may help reduce the risk of certain diseases, such as melanoma, non-melanoma skin cancer, multiple sclerosis, Alzheimer's, and Parkinson's.[9,10,11,12,13]

However, you can reap coffee's benefits only if it is:

- **Organic.** Coffee you consume should be organic and pesticide-free.

- **Fresh.** The coffee should smell and taste fresh. If your coffee does not have a pleasant aroma, it is likely rancid or of poor quality.

- **Whole bean.** Purchase coffee in whole-bean form and then grind it yourself to prevent rancidity. Pre-ground coffee may be rancid by the time you brew it.

- **Dark roast.** It's often the case that foods with the darkest pigments also offer the most robust benefits to health, and dark roast coffee, such as French roast or the beans used to make espresso or Turkish coffee, may be no exception. Research published in 2011 in *Molecular Nutrition & Food Research* found that dark roast coffee restored blood levels of the antioxidants vitamin E and glutathione more effectively than light roast coffee did.[14] The dark roast also led to a significant body weight reduction in pre-obese

volunteers, whereas the light roast did not.

- **Unsweetened.** Drink your coffee without sugar, which will spike your insulin levels and potentially lead to insulin resistance. If you really can't drink your coffee without any sweeteners, try stevia.

You can also make what's known as "keto coffee" by adding a tablespoon of organic, grass-fed butter or ghee and a tablespoon of MCT oil to make your morning coffee an efficient delivery system for healthy fats.

Further, if you use a drip coffeemaker, be sure to buy unbleached filters. The bright-white ones, which most people use, are chlorine bleached, and some of this chlorine will be extracted from the filter during the brewing process. They are also full of dangerous disinfection by-products like dioxin. (Be sure that the brand you buy is actually unbleached and not just colored brown to make you think you're buying a better product.)

To get the therapeutic benefits of coffee, drink just one cup of coffee or one shot of espresso in the morning. That's it for the day. If you exercise in the morning, have your coffee prior to your workout, not after.

Please remember that coffee should not be consumed when you are pregnant, as it may create a wide range of problems for your baby. Also, if you have high blood pressure, insomnia, or anxiety or are sensitive to the effects of caffeine, then it might be better to skip this beverage and opt for green tea or pure water instead.

SUPPLEMENT WISELY

Since the release of my book *Fat for Fuel*, my customer service team has received many inquiries regarding my recommendations for supplements; due to time and space constraints, I didn't fully outline a supplementation plan in that book.

As evidenced by the information and recipes included in this book, my primary recommendation for how to receive your nutrients is to consume primarily whole, organic food to promote fat-burning instead of using glucose as your primary source of fuel.

It's important to keep in mind that the word *supplemental* means "in addition to." So nutrients consumed in pill form should not be your primary means of providing your body the vitamins, minerals, and enzymes it needs for optimal health. Using supplements to supply all of your nutrient needs is a short-sighted and potentially dangerous strategy; food sources of nutrients are more balanced and far less likely to cause side effects.

Having said that, there are clearly many common nutrient deficiencies where the benefits of adding a supplement to your regimen far outweigh any risk to consider adding to your regimen.

Also, keep in mind that logging all your food into Cronometer helps you identify major nutrient deficiencies, and this information can certainly help guide your decisions regarding supplements.

KRILL OIL

The most important food nutrient you can consume is the essential omega-3 fatty acid DHA, which is so vital that it is the only fatty acid your body simply won't burn for fuel, unless you are starving. It is far too precious for burning, and it is stored in your cell membranes. My primary recommendation for DHA is that you get it from healthy seafood. I personally alternate between sardines, fish roe, and shrimp nearly every day. If you are eating large amounts of seafood like this, then there is simply no reason to take a DHA supplement, whether it be krill, fish oil, or DHA from algae. If you aren't sure you are eating enough healthy seafood, then I would encourage you to get an omega-3 index test, which you can buy on my website (go to shop.mercola.com and search for "vitamin D and omega 3 testing kit"), and it will let you know if you need to supplement.

Krill oil is a potent source of DHA. It is also a good source of astaxanthin, one of the most effective antioxidants on the planet, making krill oil highly resistant to oxidation.

Krill are tiny, shrimplike creatures that live in massive numbers in cold waters, such as the oceans off Antarctica. Please be assured that consuming krill oil won't threaten their population; they make up the largest biomass in the world, and harvesting of krill is carefully regulated by the Marine Stewardship Council (MSC) to avoid overfishing. Only 1 to 2 percent of the total krill biomass is harvested each year.

Krill oil is a far better alternative than fish oil supplements, which also contain omega-3 fats, because fish oil has a weak antioxidant content; unlike krill, it has no naturally occurring astaxanthin. It also has a high potential to be contaminated by mercury and other toxins and is very susceptible to spoilage.

Additionally, the fish that are used to make fish oil are very prone to mercury and other heavy metal contamination, courtesy of widespread water pollution. Antarctic krill are not prone to this contamination because they are harvested from cleaner waters, and because they feed on phytoplankton and not other contaminated fish.

In fact, a 2011 study published in the journal *Lipids* showed that krill oil is as much as 48 times more potent than fish oil, meaning you need to consume less of it than fish oil to get the same benefits.[1]

Benefits: Krill oil offers support for healthy joints, brain and nervous system function and development, the immune system, and overall mood. It helps maintain blood sugar and cholesterol levels already in the normal range. Supplementing with krill oil can help balance your omega-6:3 ratio.

Buying guidelines: When selecting a krill oil supplement, keep the following factors in mind:

- Make sure it's made from Antarctic krill, as this is by far the most abundant.

- Verify that the maker has a valid sustainability certification from the MSC, which ensures the krill were harvested in compliance with international conservation standards.

- The krill oil should be cold-processed to preserve its biological benefits. Make sure hexane is not used to extract the oil from the krill. Unfortunately, some of the most popular krill oils on the market use this dangerous chemical agent.

- The oil should also be free of heavy metals, PCBs, dioxins, and other contaminants.

- Hard capsules are preferable to softgels because the latter allow more oxygen to reach the contents, which promotes oxidization (i.e., hastens rancidity). In the absence of oxygen, no oxidation can take place. Even though krill oil contains astaxanthin, which significantly decreases oxidation, hard capsules add additional protection, assuring maximum freshness and effectiveness.

Dosage information: Aim for about 1 gram (1,000 mg) per day, according to dosage information on the label.

DETOX MINERALS: MAGNESIUM, SELENIUM, ZINC, AND IODINE

Virtually everyone living in the 21st century has a toxic load as a result of the more than 80,000 chemicals we are exposed to. For example, for virtually a century the automobile contaminated our environment with massive amounts of lead that was added to gasoline to prevent engines from knocking and that still remains in the soil. Even though it was stopped nearly 50 years ago, the lead has been replaced with thallium, another toxic metal that is added to gasoline in order to reduce engine knocking.

If you are deficient in minerals, your body will be seriously limited in its ability to remove these toxins. Detox is a very complex topic, far beyond the scope of a cookbook, but this is the primary justification for recommending magnesium, selenium, zinc, and iodine. I have one of the healthiest lifestyles of anyone I know, and these are the minerals I take. It is highly likely you will also benefit from them.

Magnesium

Magnesium is a mineral used by every organ in your body, especially your heart, muscles, and kidneys. In fact, researchers have now detected 3,751 magnesium-binding sites on human proteins,[2] indicating that its role in human health and disease may be vastly greater than originally thought.

It's quite possible to be deficient and not know it, which is why magnesium deficiency has been dubbed the "invisible deficiency." By some estimates, up to 80 percent of Americans are not getting enough magnesium. If you suffer from unexplained fatigue or weakness, abnormal heart rhythms, or even muscle spasms and eye twitches, low levels of magnesium could be to blame.

Seaweed and green leafy vegetables like spinach and Swiss chard are excellent sources of magnesium, as are pumpkin, sunflower, and sesame seeds and avocados.

However, most foods grown today are deficient in magnesium and other minerals, so getting enough isn't simply a matter of eating magnesium-rich foods (although this *is* important too). Herbicides, like glyphosate, block the uptake and utilization of minerals in so many foods grown today. As a result, it can be quite difficult to find truly magnesium-rich foods. Cooking and processing further deplete this mineral. For these reasons, it can be helpful to take a supplement.

Benefits: Magnesium plays a role in your body's detoxification processes, making it important in helping to prevent damage from environmental chemicals, heavy metals, and other toxins. Magnesium also plays a vital role in muscle and nerve function, creating energy in your body by activating adenosine triphosphate (ATP). Additionally, it helps to digest proteins, carbohydrates, and fats and acts as a precursor to neurotransmitters like serotonin.

Buying guidelines: Because magnesium must be bound to another substance, there's a wide variety of magnesium supplements on the market.

The substance used in any given compound can affect the absorption and bioavailability of the magnesium and may provide slightly different, or targeted, health benefits. Magnesium threonate and magnesium citrate are two of the best sources, as they seem to penetrate cell membranes, including your mitochondria, which results in higher energy levels. Additionally, they penetrate the blood-brain barrier—the semipermeable network of blood vessels that separates the brain from the blood of the circulatory system in a protective measure—and seem to do wonders in treating and preventing dementia and improving memory.

Whatever supplement you choose, be sure to avoid any containing magnesium stearate, a common but potentially hazardous additive.

Another way to improve your magnesium status is to take regular Epsom salt baths or footbaths. Epsom salt is a magnesium sulfate that your skin can absorb into your body. Magnesium oil can also be used for topical application and absorption.

Dosage information: Start off with doses around 150 mg of magnesium threonate or citrate a day, then increase from there. It would be wise to work your intake of elemental magnesium up to 500 to 800 mg daily to help mitigate EMF effect. Use the "bowel test" to determine when you reach your personal threshold of too much magnesium, then back off that dose. In other words, supplement until your stools become loose, then back down from that dose until your stools are regular. Whatever amount you take in that is above your body's optimal amount will simply be flushed away.

Selenium

Selenium is a trace element a Swedish chemist, Baron Jöns Jacob Berzelius, discovered almost 200 years ago. Today, scientists recognize it as an essential mineral for human health, with potent anti-inflammatory, antiviral, and anticancer properties. It raises your white blood cell count so you're more able to resist infections.

Benefits: At the cellular level, selenium is an active component of glutathione peroxidase, an enzyme that converts hydrogen peroxide to water. Glutathione peroxidase has potent antioxidant properties and serves as a first line of defense against the buildup of harmful free radicals in your cells.

Selenium also plays an important role in the prevention of cancer. One of the reasons people get cancer is because of excessive free radical production. By reducing free radicals, selenium helps reduce your risk of cancer.

Buying guidelines: If you opt for a supplement, make sure to get the high-selenium yeast form, such as SelenoExcell, which is

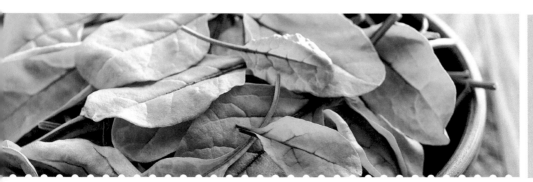

the scientifically tested and most recommended version.

Dosage information: Selenium is needed in very small, microgram amounts (a microgram is a thousandth of a milligram). More is not better here, as toxicity can become an issue. For cancer prevention, the recommended level is 200 mcg per day. Many studies have used as much as 400 mcg per day without ill effect. However, since most of the research supports the use of 200 mcg per day and shows no significant benefits at higher amounts, I don't recommend exceeding 200 mcg per day.

If you enjoy eating Brazil nuts, eating about two to three of them per day will typically be sufficient.

Zinc

Zinc is an essential trace mineral, probably most widely known for the integral role it plays in your immune system and the prevention and treatment of the common cold. Aside from iron, zinc is the most common mineral found in your body, necessary for the function of every one of your cells.

However, while zinc is essential, your body does not store it, so it is important you get enough every day. The RDA for zinc is about 11 milligrams (mg) per day for adult men and 8 mg for women. If you are lactating or pregnant, you need about 3 mg more. For children, 4- to 8-year-olds need about 5 mg, 9- to 13-year-olds need 8 mg, and infants need only about 3 mg.

It's not easy to get zinc strictly from food, because even under the best circumstances your body may absorb only 20 percent to 40 percent of the zinc in your food.[3]

Benefits: Zinc is used in the production of white blood cells, helping your body fight infection, and plays a key role in regulating the way your heart muscle uses calcium to trigger the electrical stimulus responsible for your heartbeat. It's also one of the building blocks for approximately 3,000 proteins and 200 enzymes in your body and plays a role in protecting your DNA.

Buying guidelines: If you choose to use a supplement, ensure it is from a reputable company using best-practice, quality assurance methods. Independent verification of the raw materials is vital to confirm quality and ensure that the product is free of lead and other heavy metals. The supplement should contain several different types of zinc, such as gluconate, citrate, and chelate.

Dosage information: Unless your clinician recommends otherwise, don't go above 40 milligrams (mg) per day.

It's important to keep in mind that regularly getting too much zinc can be just as hazardous as getting too little, as it can interfere with your body's ability to absorb other minerals, especially copper.

Iodine

Iodine is necessary for your thyroid, which in turn produces hormones crucial for metabolism and energy regulation. Iodine is also used by many other parts of the body, including breasts, skin, salivary glands, stomach, pancreas, brain, cerebral spinal fluid, and thymus.

Iodine deficiency in any of these tissues will lead to dysfunction of that tissue. Hence the following symptoms could provide clues that you're not getting enough iodine in your diet.

- Salivary glands: inability to produce saliva, leading to dry mouth

- Skin: dryness and lack of sweating

- Brain: reduced alertness and lowered IQ

- Muscles: nodules, scar tissue, pain, fibrosis, and fibromyalgia

Benefits: In addition to its vital role in thyroid regulation, iodine has several important functions in your body: stabilizing metabolism and body weight, supporting brain development in children, supporting fertility, optimizing the immune system (iodine is a potent antibacterial, antiparasitic, antiviral, and anticancer agent), and stimulating apoptosis, the process by which defective cells, such as cancer cells, self-destruct.

Buying guidelines: Toxin-free sea vegetables and spirulina are likely the ideal natural sources from which to obtain your iodine. Just make sure that these are harvested from uncontaminated waters (especially if you're pregnant!), and be careful not to overdo it. Sea vegetables also provide valuable minerals and even modulate your gut flora, altering estrogen metabolism and lowering your risk of breast cancer.[4] (One study found that consuming a sheet of nori a day may cut a woman's risk of breast cancer in half.[5])

Other seafood, such as wild-caught scallops, sardines, salmon, and shrimp, contain iodine as well, as do raw milk, eggs, and even strawberries.

Dosage information: The dose of sea vegetables is about 5 grams a day or about one ounce per week. You can also use iodine supplements. If you need to replace iodine stores, then a few weeks to a few months of 10 mg per day is fine, but long-term maintenance doses are closer to 2.5 mg per day.

ASTAXANTHIN

Astaxanthin is a highly effective antioxidant—perhaps the most potent biological antioxidant we know of. There are only two natural astaxanthin sources: the microalgae *Haematococcus pluvialis*, which produce it, and the sea creatures that consume the algae, such as salmon and krill. When *H. pluvialis*'s water supply dries up, it has a survival mechanism to protect itself from intense sunlight, ultraviolet radiation, and low nutrition, and it's this survival mechanism that lends astaxanthin its power to protect your cells from free radicals. In addition, it can cross the blood-brain and blood-retinal barriers, a feat that can't be claimed by most antioxidants.

Benefits: Astaxanthin helps in supporting your eyes, brain, and immune and cardiovascular systems. It also helps lower your blood sugar levels, mitigating the risk of diseases linked to high blood sugar levels. It can enhance your endurance, workout performance, and recovery as well.

This antioxidant also aids in healing injuries to the spinal cord and nervous system, lessening inflammation from all causes, lowering oxidative damage to DNA, relieving indigestion and reflux, preventing sunburn, and protecting your body from radiation.

Buying guidelines: If you take a krill oil supplement too, it will naturally contain astaxanthin; check the label to see how much you're already getting with that before you buy an astaxanthin supplement. If you only need a small amount of astaxanthin to get to

2 mg (the recommended starting dose; see "dosage information" below for more info), you won't want a supplement that delivers 1 mg per capsule.

Dosage information: Start with 4 mg per day and work your way up to about 12 mg per day, or more if you're an athlete or suffering from chronic inflammation and need additional antioxidant support. If you are on a krill oil supplement, which naturally contains astaxanthin, take that into consideration. Different krill products have different concentrations of astaxanthin, so check your label. Another factor to keep in mind is that astaxanthin is a fat-soluble supplement. So unless you take it with a small amount of fat, your body won't absorb it well. Butter, coconut oil, or eggs would be ideal complements to ensure optimal absorption.

PROBIOTICS

The more I study health, the more I have come to appreciate how crucially important your microbiome is. Most people, including many physicians, do not realize that 80 percent of your immune system is located in your digestive system, making a healthy gut a major focal point for maintaining optimal health.

Furthermore, your gut is quite literally your second brain: it originates from the same type of tissue as your brain! During fetal development, one part turns into your central nervous system, while the other develops into your enteric nervous system (which innervates the gastrointestinal tract). These two systems are connected via the vagus nerve, the tenth cranial nerve that runs from your brain stem down to your abdomen. Hence your gut and your brain work in tandem, each influencing the other. And this is why your intestinal health can have such a profound influence on your mental health, and vice versa.

The ideal way to optimize your gut flora is to exclude all sugars and processed foods, which inhibit beneficial bacteria by nourishing pathogenic bacteria. The next step would be to add high-quality, unpasteurized, fermented foods to your diet; eating them daily is the ideal way to boost the population of friendly bacteria. If you are regularly eating fermented foods, then you likely will have little to no benefit from a probiotic supplement.

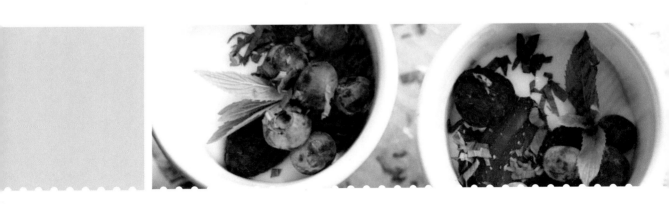

However, if you don't enjoy the taste of fermented foods or can't quite develop a daily habit of eating them, then adding a daily probiotic supplement to your regimen makes sense. It will help you maintain a robust population of health-promoting friendly bacteria and improve health in multiple ways.

Benefits: Probiotic supplements help seed a healthy population of friendly bacteria that, once established, do the following:

- Assist in the elimination of toxins
- Aid in food digestion and absorption of nutrients
- Enhance synthesis of B vitamins
- Improve calcium absorption
- Help balance intestinal microflora
- Promote vaginal health in women
- Support the immune system
- Help to mitigate mental health issues, such as anxiety and depression

Buying guidelines: I recommend looking for a probiotic supplement that fulfills the following criteria, to ensure quality and efficacy:

- The bacteria strains in the product must be able to survive your stomach acid and bile so that they reach your intestines alive in adequate numbers (you can determine this by reading the packaging carefully, or by visiting the website or calling the manufacturer—they should be testing the supplements to determine viability).

- The bacteria strains must have health-promoting features (you can do an Internet search on the specific strains listed in the ingredients).

- The probiotic activity must be guaranteed throughout the entire production process, storage period, and shelf life of the product (again, you can find this by reading the packaging or by visiting the website or calling the manufacturer).

Through my years of clinical practice, I've found that no single probiotic supplement works for everyone. The key here is to identify a high-quality, multi-strain, high-potency supplement. We sell one on Mercola.com, but other companies also sell them.

Dosage information: Follow the directions on the bottle, as dosage varies by manufacturer.

UBIQUINOL

Ubiquinol is the reduced and more bioavailable form of coenzyme Q10 (CoQ10), which is used for energy production by every cell in your body. It is absolutely vital that anyone who is on a statin or has heart disease take this on a daily basis. It is optional for others, but the older you are, the more likely you will benefit as your body makes less as you age.

So if you are interested in slowing your aging process, this would be a wise choice for you.

Ubiquinol is a lipid-soluble (fat-soluble) antioxidant, meaning it helps prevent cellular damage from free radicals in the lipid portions of your body, such as your cell membranes and in your mitochondria. It's one of the very few antioxidants that are fat-soluble, which makes it extremely valuable to your health. You see, when your mitochondria produce energy within your cells, that process produces free radical by-products. One of the functions of ubiquinol is to mop up those by-products. When ubiquinol is lacking, the by-products remain and begin damaging the cell.

You make your own ubiquinol, but by the time you hit the age of 30, it begins to decline. Another factor is the class of cholesterol-lowering drugs known as statins. In addition to hindering the body's production of cholesterol, statins also impair your production of ubiquinol, and the resulting depletion can have very severe consequences. When you reduce your ubiquinol levels, the conversion of your food to energy becomes less efficient, which leads to lower energy, fatigue, and muscle pain. This becomes especially problematic when you consider that at least one in four American adults over the age of 40 is currently taking a statin drug, and that number is expected to reach one in three.

Benefits: Ubiquinol works to improve your cardiovascular system, jump-start your body's energy and stamina levels, reduce the visible signs of aging, act as an antioxidant and protect your body from free radicals, maintain normal blood pressure levels and promote healthy blood circulation, boost your immune system, support your nervous system, and stimulate an active mind.

Dosage guidelines: Dosing requirements will vary depending on your individual situation and needs, but some general guidelines can still be useful. As a general rule, the sicker you are, the more you need. If you're just starting out with ubiquinol, start with 200 to 300 mg per day. Within three weeks, your plasma levels will typically plateau to their optimum level. After that, you can go down to a 100 mg/day maintenance dose. This dose is typically sufficient for healthy people. If you have an active lifestyle, exercise a lot, or are under a lot of stress due to your job or life in general, you may want to increase your dose to 200 to 300 mg/day.

If you're on a statin drug, you *must* take at least 100 mg of ubiquinol per day, or more. To address heart failure and/or other significant heart problems, you may need around 350 mg per day or more. Ideally, you'll want to work with your physician to ascertain your ideal dose. Your doctor can do a blood test to measure your CoQ10 levels, which would tell you whether your dose is high enough to keep you within a healthy range.

If you're taking one of the higher doses, split it up and take it two or three times a day, rather than all at once; this will result in higher blood levels.

MULTIVITAMINS

If you are avoiding all processed foods, limiting sugar, and eating organic whole foods at all times, then it is not likely you will benefit from a multivitamin. I personally don't take one but recognize many are unable to follow this type of eating plan for a wide variety of reasons. If you are one of those people, then it would make sense to give yourself some insurance with a high-quality multivitamin.

Multivitamins have been the subject of some conflicting reports of efficacy, but statistics show that one-third of Americans today take multivitamins, with the number rising to about 40 percent among older Americans. And a large body of research indicates that multivitamins are actually beneficial for the average American.

One study of nearly 9,000 adults followed the participants for nearly two decades to see whether or not multivitamin use played a role in heart health. Among women, but not men, taking multivitamin-mineral supplements for at least three years was associated with a 35 percent lower risk of dying from heart disease.[6] This doesn't prove cause and effect, and the fact that people who take multivitamins often tend to lead healthier lifestyles overall could account for the heart benefits. Still, the researchers accounted for many other heart risk factors, such as weight, blood pressure, blood sugar control, education, and alcohol use, and the association still remained.

It's important to note that the lowered risk of illnesses was seen after about three years of regular multivitamin use. So not only are multivitamins not complete solutions, they are also not quick fixes. For your health, it pays to think long term, and multivitamin use can help you do that.

Multivitamins also save on health care costs. A report by the Council for Responsible Nutrition (CRN) says that $11 billion could be saved *each year* in U.S. health care costs if people would take supplements for prevention.

Benefits: Multivitamin use is associated with a reduced risk of heart disease, diabetes-related heart disease, age-related eye disease, and osteoporosis.

These benefits extend not only to the person taking the multivitamin, but also to the next generation. While it is important for women who are pregnant or want to become pregnant to take a high-quality multivitamin, men's health at time of conception may also be vital to delivering a healthy child.

Fifty percent of pregnancies are not planned, so it is important we educate our young adults about the value of multivitamins. This age group is typically not the most interested in obtaining proper nutrition, and I feel it is absolutely critical for the future generations that all young men and women consider a high-quality multivitamin.

Buying guidelines: When selecting a high-quality multivitamin, be sure it is as close as possible to its natural (whole food) form and follows industry standards for quality assurance, including ISO 9001, ISO 17025, and Good Manufacturing Processes (GMP) certifications.

One caveat: Men of all ages and postmenopausal women should choose a brand that does not include iron. Too much iron is toxic, and the body doesn't have any means of excreting excess iron except for menstruation. So please avoid any iron supplements unless your child needs them, or you are a premenopausal woman, or you have been told by your physician that you are iron deficient. Iron toxicity is a very serious and common problem, so please be careful.

Dosage information: Varies greatly from multivitamin to multivitamin; check labels for guidance.

CHOOSE THE RIGHT COOKING METHODS

Cooking your food, especially at high temperatures, destroys naturally occurring enzymes. So it's not just what foods you eat, and when you eat them, that make up the total picture of how healthy your diet is; how you cook them matters too. After all, cooking is a form of chemistry. As you cook your food a chemical reaction happens, and different types of cooking produce different types of chemical reactions. This is one reason why foods that are baked in the oven will taste different from those that are steamed, sautéed on the stove, or grilled over an open flame.

How you prepare the food before you cook it matters as well. The addition of spices and marinades before you ever turn on a burner changes the chemicals present during the cooking process and therefore the chemical reactions occurring while you cook. The type of knife you use to cut your meat or vegetables in preparation for cooking also makes a difference.

In this chapter, I'll share some of my favorite tips for cooking your healthy food, and some might surprise you.

1. TAKE CARE WHEN GRILLING

Eighty percent of U.S. households own a grill or smoker and have used it in the past year. Grilling gives a distinctive flavor to food and is a nice way to spend time outdoors with family and friends. However, grilling also creates changes in food that could potentially produce cancer-causing chemicals. Specifically, grilling has been show to produce:

- **Heterocyclic Amines (HCAs).** These chemicals are formed in muscle meat when it's cooked at high temperatures. Even cooking at high temperatures over the stove can cause the formation of HCAs.[1] In experiments with laboratory animals, HCAs have been shown to be mutagenic. This means they cause changes to the lab animals' DNA. When HCAs were fed to rodents, they developed cancer in multiple organs, including the colon, breast, and prostate.[2]

The amount of HCAs present depends on the type of meat, how well done it is, and the temperature used to cook the meat. For example, researchers have found that well-done meat has three and a half times more HCAs than medium-rare meat and that fried pork has more than fried beef or fried chicken.[3]

- **Advanced Glycation End Products (AGEs).** AGEs, also known as glycotoxins, are highly oxidant compounds linked to increased inflammation and oxidation stress in your body.[4] AGEs are present in food before it is cooked; grilling appears to create more of them. Study findings indicate that dry heat from grilling or broiling may increase the formation of AGEs tenfold to a hundredfold, compared with uncooked foods.

    The formation of AGEs in your body is a normal part of metabolism. The addition of more AGEs from the food you eat increases the likelihood that the amount of circulating AGEs will become pathogenic. Your body does not get rid of or digest these end products easily. Instead, they are stored in your organs and over time cause damage.

    Multiple studies have found mice that ate diets rich in AGEs suffered from diabetes, diabetic tissue damage, atherosclerosis, and slow wound healing.[5,6,7,8] Mice fed diets low in AGEs experienced significantly less risk of the same health issues.

    Animal meat, such as beef and chicken, is generally rich in AGEs. Lamb has less than other meats, as do eggs.[9] Researchers found a reduction in the formation of new AGEs in meat cooked with moist heat, with shorter cooking times, at lower temperatures, and with acidic ingredients.[10]

- **Polycyclic Aromatic Hydrocarbons (PAHs).** PAHs don't originate in meat but rather in the wood, gas, or coal you use for your grill fire. They are also formed when fat from meat drips on the grill and creates smoke. The compound is in the smoke and is deposited on anything it touches. This means that PAHs will cling to the meat and your clothing and that you will inhale them as you stand over the grill. This is troublesome because exposure to PAHs is known to cause skin, liver, and stomach cancers in lab animals.[11]

    What's worse, when the PAHs from the swoke mingle with the nitrogen from the meat you're cooking, nitrated PAHs (NPAHs) are formed. These are even more carcinogenic.

While the health dangers of grilling are serious, you don't need to post your grill on Craigslist just yet, however. Here are a few ways to reduce your exposure to HCAs, AGEs, and PAHs when grilling food:

- **Choose accompaniments wisely.** The following foods have been found to help reduce the amount of HCAs and AGEs produced when grilling: cherries, garlic, onion, rosemary, thyme, virgin olive oil, mustard, cloves, cider vinegar, cinnamon, oregano, black pepper, paprika, and ginger.[12] Add them to your grass-fed burger patties, or use them in a rub to decrease the risks associated with this popular cooking method.

- **Trim the fat when grilling.** Remove the skin from chicken, trim the fat from steaks, choose leaner cuts of meat for the grill, and skip the fatty sausage and ribs altogether.

- **Skip the char.** Those crisscross grill marks you work to achieve are just another indication of a buildup of AGEs and HCAs. Forget the crisscrosses. Instead, flip the meat frequently at a lower temperature or cook it using indirect heat (not directly over the flame). Remove any burned or charred meat before eating.

- **Avoid overcooking.** To reduce the amount of HCAs and AGEs in your grilled food, choose a medium-cooked meat over one that's well done. For safety, use a meat thermometer to check the temperature of the meat. Steak should be cooked to 145 degrees Fahrenheit (F), hamburgers to 160 degrees F, and chicken to 165 degrees F. Place the thermometer in the center of the meat, away from bone, fat, or gristle.

- **Use marinades and rubs.** A tasty marinade helps improve your cooking in a number of ways. The marinade reduces the amount of fat dripping into the grill, and thus the amount of smoke and PAHs. Acidic marinades reduce the amount of HCAs produced when cooking. A mixture of one part lemon juice to two parts onion and garlic was found to reduce the production of HCAs in grilling by up to 70 percent.[13]

- **Avoid barbecue sauces.** Sauces made with tomato and/or sugars will double and sometimes triple your ingestion of toxic chemicals after just 15 minutes of cooking.[14] The sugar content can also impair your transition to burning fat.

- **Precook your meat.** Precooking indoors removes some of the fat that may drip into the flame and reduces the cooking time on the grill, thereby also reducing the amount of time the food is exposed to toxins. Less time at high heat reduces the number of AGEs developed in the meat during cooking.

2. DON'T MICROWAVE YOUR FOOD

It's really best not to use a microwave at all. You can easily substitute a toaster oven or a steam convection oven about the same size as a microwave that will heat food nearly as quickly without the dangerous side effects.

By now, you probably know that what you eat has a profound impact on your health. The mantra "You are what you eat" is really true. But you need to consider not only what you buy, but also how you cook it. When it comes to microwave ovens, the price for convenience is to compromise your health.

Microwave ovens can produce carcinogenic toxins in more ways than one. When plastic is heated, toxic chemicals like BPA and phthalates can leach out of the containers or covers, contaminating your food with endocrine and hormone disruptors. A paper published in 1990 reported the leakage of many toxic chemicals from the packaging of common microwavable foods, including pizzas, chips, and popcorn. Chemicals included polyethylene terepthalate (PET) and well-documented carcinogens like dioxin, benzene, toluene, and xylene.

How Microwaves Damage Your Health

You might not be aware of this, but microwave ovens operate on gigahertz frequencies very similar to most 4G cellular networks. So, the dangers and the justifications of why you should avoid both are identical.

New research from Dr. Martin Pall has provided us with the mechanism of how this low-level nonthermal microwave exposure causes biological harm. It has to do with voltage gated calcium channels (VGCCs) that are embedded in the cell membranes. He determined this by evaluating over two dozen studies showing you can radically reduce biological microwave damage using calcium channel blockers.

This explains why the argument that the microwave radiation is not high enough to cause thermal damage is fatally flawed. The statement is partially correct, as the radiation does not cause thermal damage. However, it causes massive biological damage.

So just how does it cause damage? Well, once the VGCCs are activated by microwaves, about one million calcium ions per second, these ions then stimulate the release of nitric oxide, which combines with superoxide to

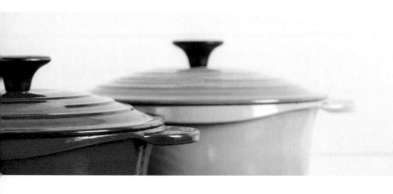

form peroxynitrate. These peroxynitrates then create hydroxyl free radicals, the most destructive free radicals known to man, which decimate mitochondrial and nuclear DNA, membranes, and proteins that lead to mitochondrial dysfunction, the core of most chronic disease.

Pall has calculated that these VGCCs are over 7 million times more sensitive to microwave radiation than the charged particles inside and outside the cell, which means the currently established safety standards are off by a factor of over 7 *million*.

Failure to realize this and take steps to minimize exposure will not only damage your DNA and increase your risk of most chronic illness; it will also seriously impair your body's ability to remove toxins, and significantly impair your immune response to address the large variety of pathogenic infectious assaults you regularly encounter, especially parasites.

So, every time you turn on your microwave oven, you are exposing yourself to microwave radiation densities thousands of times higher than your cell phone. This is the primary reason why I strongly advise removing the microwave from your home.[15, 16, 17]

Breaking Free of Your Microwave: A Few Basic Tips

Hopefully, I have provided you with enough compelling information to stop using your microwave. If real estate in your kitchen is at a premium, your microwave should probably be the first thing to go. Contrary to popular belief, you can survive quite well without it. I tossed mine out last year and replaced it with a similar-sized steam convection oven that cooks nearly as quickly as a microwave but more safely. You can also:

- **Plan ahead.** Take your dinner out of the freezer in the morning, or the night before, so you don't end up having to scramble to defrost a five-pound chunk of beef two hours before dinnertime.

- **Make soups and stews in bulk**, then freeze them in gallon-size freezer bags or other containers. An hour before mealtime, just take one out and defrost it in a sink of water until it's thawed enough to slip into a pot, then reheat it on the stove.

- **Use a toaster oven instead.** A toaster oven makes a *great* faux microwave for heating up leftovers! Keep it at a low temperature, about 200 degrees F, and gently warm a plate of food over the course of 10 to 15 minutes. Another great alternative is a convection oven, as I mentioned above.

3. CHOOSE THE RIGHT POTS AND PANS

I know how alluring the convenience of nonstick cookware is, but these pots and pans simply leach too many chemicals when heated to be wise choices. The poly- and perfluoroalkyl substances (PFAS) used to create these surfaces are toxic and highly persistent, both in your body and in the environment.

When heated, a nonstick cookware surface such as Teflon becomes a source of perfluorooctanoic acid (PFOA), a long-chain perfluorinated chemical linked to a range of health problems, including thyroid disease, infertility in women, and organ damage and developmental and reproductive problems in lab animals.

The U.S. Environmental Protection Agency (EPA) has also ruled that perfluorinated compounds (PFCs) are "likely carcinogens."

In studies of heated nonstick pans on conventional stovetops, commissioned by the consumer watchdog organization Environmental Working Group (EWG), it only took *two to five minutes* of heating to reach temperatures at which dangerous toxins were produced.[18]

According to the EWG, studies conducted by DuPont's own scientists revealed that when its nonstick Teflon cookware is heated it breaks down into 15 types of toxic gases and particles.[19] Despite that, these chemicals are still used in a wide array of household products.

While some will recommend using aluminum, stainless steel, and copper cookware, I don't. Aluminum is a strongly suspected causal factor in Alzheimer's disease. And stainless steel has alloys containing nickel (as well as chromium, molybdenum, and carbon), which is a particularly important consideration for those with nickel allergies. Copper cookware is also not recommended because most copper pans come lined with other metals, creating the same concerns as with stainless steel pots and pans.

Healthier options include ceramic and enameled cast-iron cookware, both of which are durable, easy to clean (even the toughest cooked-on foods can be wiped away after soaking in warm water), and completely inert, which means they won't release any harmful chemicals. I don't recommend regular cast-iron pans, as they leach iron into the foods cooked in them; as I discussed on page 64, excess iron can become a hazard to your health.

One type of pot that can be an ideal option is a pressure cooker. In addition to shaving hours off cooking times, using a pressure cooker is also one of the most effective ways to destroy harmful lectins.[20]

Pressure cooking, especially in the newer pressure cookers, destroys lectins in food and may also preserve more nutrients than other cooking methods. In one study, cooking spinach and amaranth in a pressure cooker was the best method to preserve the beta-carotene and ascorbic acid in the food.[21] A 2007 study found that broccoli cooked in a pressure cooker maintained 90 percent of its vitamin C, significantly more than when it was steamed or boiled.

Pressure cookers require very little cooking liquid, which means there is less chance for nutrients from the food to leach into water or broth. Because the food cooks more quickly, you also have less chance of burning and developing compounds such as acrylamides. One of the best modern pressure cookers is Instant Pot.

HOW THE RIGHT KNIFE CAN ACTUALLY IMPROVE NUTRIENT CONTENT

Having the right knife can make cooking prep much easier and more enjoyable. But you may not realize that the right knife can increase the nutrients that the foods you're chopping provide your body.

There's a (relatively) new school of thought that says chopping vegetables increases the polyphenols they provide. Polyphenols are found only in plants and have several different jobs, such as providing the plant's color and protecting the plant against damage from ultraviolet radiation. If you nick or cut certain vegetables, such as celery, parsnips, and lettuce, they'll produce more polyphenols to defend against further damage. If an animal starts to eat the vegetable, for instance, the bitterness of the polyphenols may keep it from taking a second bite. In humans, chopping veggies or slicing them may make the bioactive compounds in them more bioavailable, and health benefits can be derived from synergistic combinations of phytochemicals.[22]

One study showed that, depending on the type of vegetable tissue, "wounding" (i.e., cutting) it may also increase its antioxidant capacity. Chopping or peeling veggies can sometimes cause them to turn brown. You've probably seen it; that first peeled potato takes on an unsightly brown shade even before you get to the second one. This phenomenon occurs due to the enzyme polyphenol oxidase breaking down the polyphenols.

Believe it or not, the knife you use can make all the difference. Iron and copper increase the browning rate, and that's what most stainless steel knives are made from, among other metals. In the cutting, your veggies get the triple whammy of oxygen and the concoction created by mixing the abovementioned metals.

Ceramic and plastic knives, on the other hand, are chemically inert, which may slow the browning process. In testing, *Cook's Illustrated* found that using a plastic knife prevented browning of lettuce for a full day longer than a metal knife or tearing by hand.[23] Ceramic knives and stainless steel knives were then tested on apples and avocados, and while neither prevented browning entirely, the avocados took visibly longer to turn brown when cut with the ceramic knife.

Rather than replacing all your knives, you can use ceramic blades to complement your other cutlery. They're best for slicing fruit, vegetables, and boneless meat, but not for frozen foods, meat with bones, or cheese (because of its tendency to stick). Nor should they be used to crush foods like garlic.

NOW GO FORTH AND PREPARE YOUR FOOD

I hope that reviewing your pots, pans, and knives will further inspire you to dive into the recipes that Pete Evans has so thoughtfully organized. Bon appétit!

IMPORTANT: REMEMBER THIS BEFORE YOU PREPARE YOUR FOOD

Please understand that just because a recipe is in this book doesn't mean it is compatible with your cyclical ketogenic diet. You will still need to weigh and enter your food in Cronometer to determine if the macronutrient ratios are consistent with the recommendations for you in *Fat for Fuel*.

Most of the recipes will be fine, but you will need to pay careful attention to your portion size to keep yourself in the cyclical ketogenic zone. And always remember that when you are in circumstances when you just won't be able to access these types of foods, you have another not frequently considered option. You can choose not to eat—or fast. If you are seriously underweight, this may not be an optimal strategy, but for most of us it is an option that will not only allow us to avoid disease causing foods but also help keep us in ketosis and optimize the function of our mitochondria.

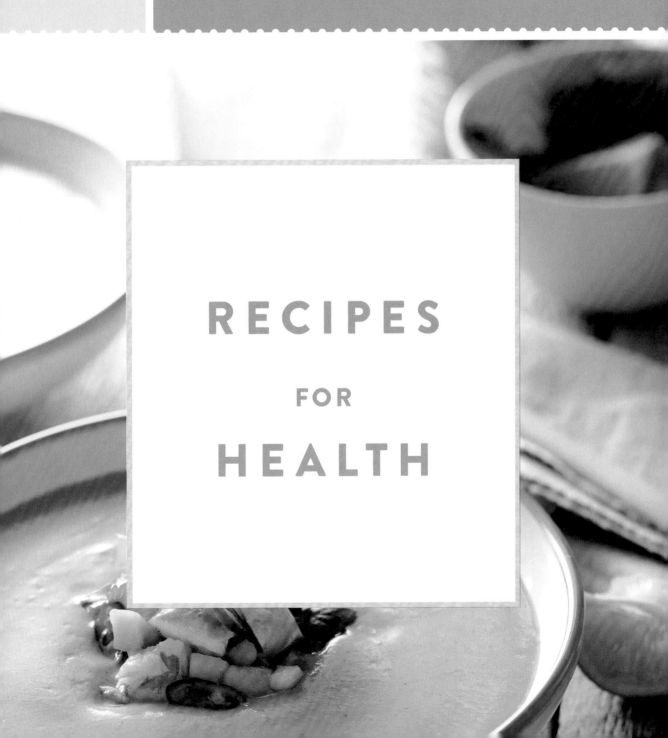

PART II

RECIPES

FOR

HEALTH

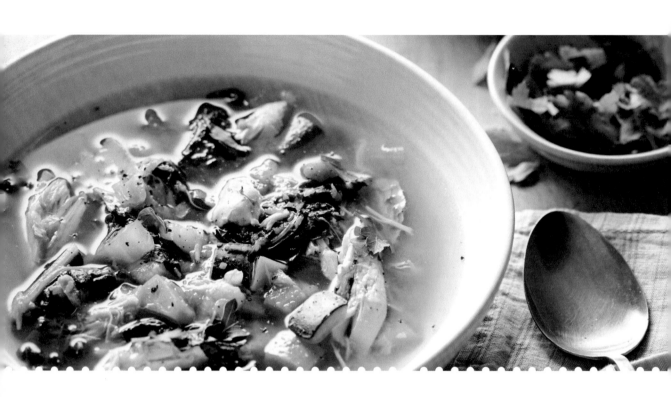

BROTHS AND SOUPS

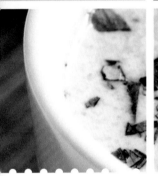
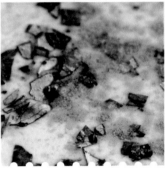
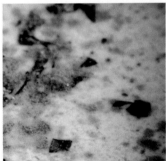
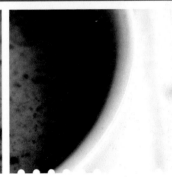

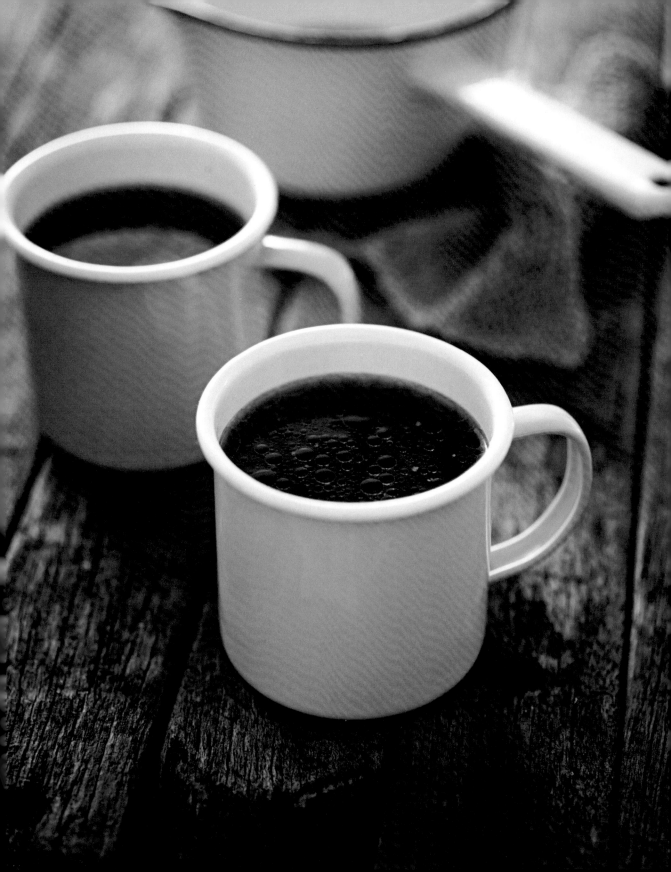

BEEF BONE BROTH

Place the beef knuckles and marrowbones in a stockpot or very large saucepan. Add the vinegar and 5 quarts of cold water, or enough to cover, and allow the mixture to stand for 1 hour.

Preheat the oven to 400°F. Put the meaty rib bones, onions, parsley, carrots, and leeks in a roasting pan and roast for 20 minutes, until well browned. Transfer to the stockpot along with the celery.

Pour the fat out of the roasting pan into a separate saucepan with 4 cups of water. Place the saucepan over high heat and bring to a simmer, stirring with a wooden spoon to break up any coagulated solids. Add this liquid to the bones and vegetables. Add additional water, if necessary, to cover the bones, but don't allow the liquid to come within ¾ inch of the rim of the stockpot because the volume increases slightly during cooking.

Bring the stock to a boil, skimming off any scum that rises to the top. Reduce the heat to low and add the thyme, peppercorns, and garlic.

Simmer the stock for a minimum of 8 hours and up to 12 hours until the broth is flavorsome and golden in color. Strain the stock through a fine-mesh sieve into a large container. Cover and cool in the refrigerator. Remove the fat that congeals at the top. Transfer to smaller, airtight containers. The stock can be stored in the refrigerator for 3 to 4 days or frozen for up to 3 months.

NOTE: The reserved fat can be used as a cooking oil for meat, poultry, and vegetables dishes.

Makes: 5 quarts

4½ lb beef knuckles and marrowbones

3 Tbsp apple cider vinegar

3½ lb meaty beef rib or neck bones

3 onions, roughly chopped

2 large handfuls flat-leaf parsley

3 carrots, roughly chopped

2 leeks (white part only), rinsed and roughly chopped

3 celery stalks, roughly chopped

6 thyme sprigs, tied together

1 tsp black peppercorns, crushed

1 garlic bulb, cut in half crosswise

BEEF BROTH WITH TURMERIC, COCONUT CREAM, AND GINGER

If you have read any of Pete's other cookbooks, you will know by now how important bone broth is for your gut and overall health. This simple beef broth comes in handy when you want something in the morning to get you through to lunchtime or when you don't want a full meal at the end of the day.

For variation, you could easily replace the beef base with a chicken, pork, or fish base. It will help you to feel wonderfully satiated. If you need or want extra fat, then add some coconut oil or bone marrow.

Serves: 3

2 cups Beef Bone Broth (see recipe, page 77)

1 Tbsp finely grated fresh ginger

½ tsp ground turmeric, plus extra to serve

1 cup coconut cream

Sea salt and freshly ground black pepper

Juice of ½ lime (optional)

1 tsp finely chopped coriander

Place the broth, ginger, turmeric, and coconut cream in a saucepan and bring to a simmer over medium heat. Cook, stirring occasionally, for 5 minutes to allow the ginger and turmeric to infuse. Season with salt and pepper. If you like your broth slightly tart, stir in lime juice to taste.

Pour the broth into mugs, sprinkle with coriander and a touch more turmeric, take a sip, and enjoy!

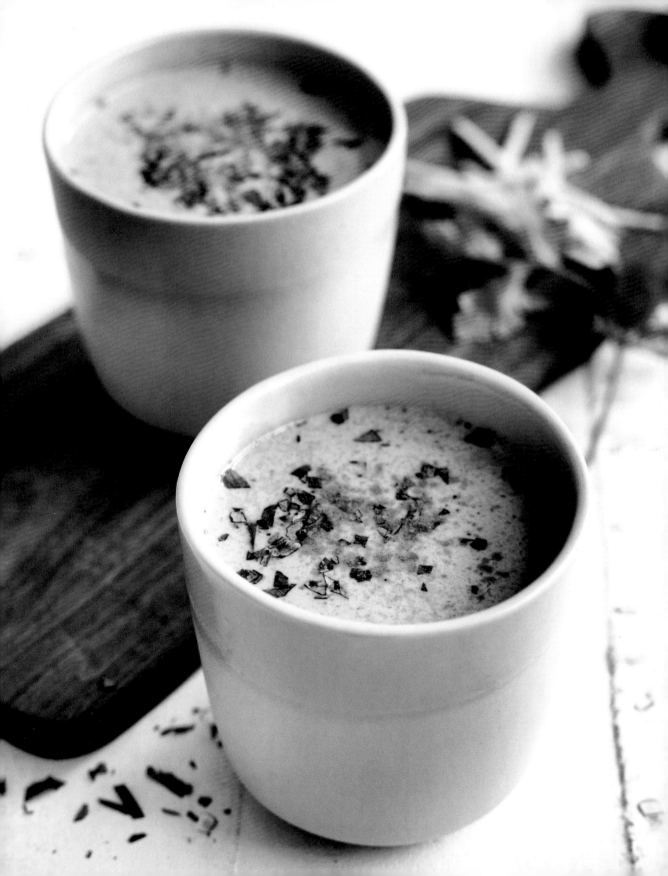

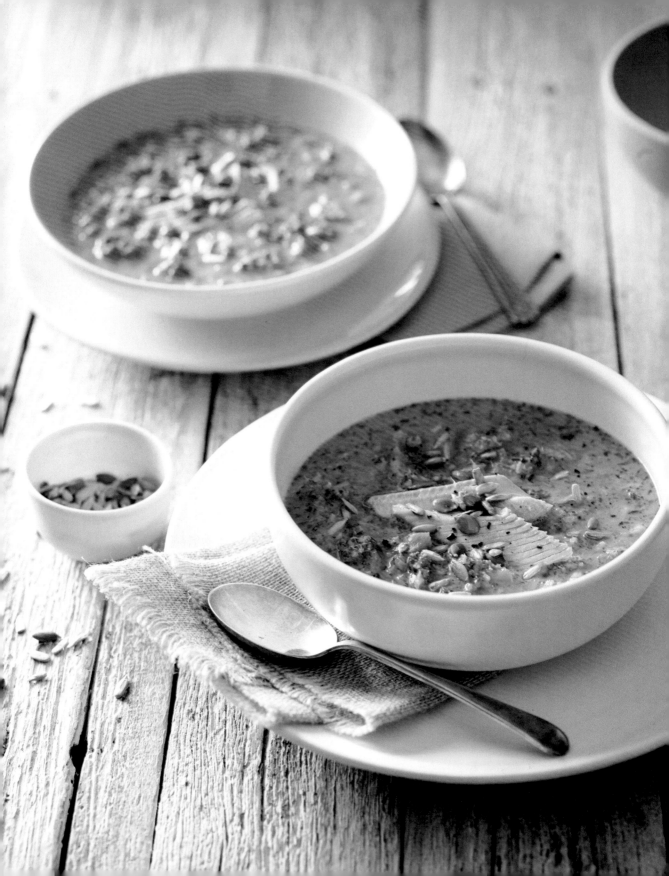

BROCCOLI SOUP WITH WILD HOT SMOKED TROUT AND ROSEMARY

Pete really loves this dish as it's such a great way to get nutrient-rich broccoli into your diet. He has teamed it with some smoked trout here, but you could just as easily fry up a little bacon or add some leftover roast chicken or cooked wild shrimp. It's also great as a chilled soup the next day for lunch, packed into a cold thermos.

Heat oil in a saucepan over medium-high heat. Add the onion and cook for 5 minutes, until translucent. Add the broccoli stalks and garlic and cook for another 5 minutes or so, until they start to brown, stirring occasionally. Add the broccoli florets, rosemary, and dill, then pour in the broth and bring to a boil. Reduce the heat to medium-low and gently simmer for 20 minutes, until the broccoli is tender. Season with salt and pepper.

Using a handheld or stick blender, blend the soup until it has a thick, chunky consistency. Ladle the soup into serving bowls, then top with the flaked trout, a sprinkle of toasted seeds, and a bit of lemon zest. Serve hot.

Serves: 4

2 Tbsp coconut oil, duck fat, tallow, or other good-quality fat

1 onion, chopped

2 heads broccoli, crowns broken into florets and stalks chopped

2 cloves garlic, minced

1 Tbsp finely chopped fresh rosemary

1 Tbsp finely chopped dill (leaves only), plus extra for garnish

3 cups Chicken Bone Broth (see recipe, page 87)

Sea salt and freshly ground black pepper

1 wild smoked rainbow trout, skin and bones removed, flesh flaked

2 Tbsp of presoaked sunflower and pumpkin seeds, toasted

Zest of 1 lemon

BROTH WITH GREENS AND BONE MARROW

If you want good fats with low-carbohydrate greens or vegetables, then it cannot get any easier than this. The addition of bone marrow gives this dish some lovely saturated fat, which is so good for us.

Serves: 4

1¾ lb center-cut beef marrowbones, cut into 1½ inch pieces, tendons trimmed (ask your butcher to do this)

Sea salt

4 cups Beef, Chicken, or Fish Bone Broth (see recipes, pages 77, 87, and 91)

½ onion, sliced

3 Swiss chard leaves, chopped

3 rainbow chard leaves, chopped

Freshly ground black pepper

1 to 2 Tbsp lemon juice

1 to 2 pinches chili flakes (optional)

Preheat the oven to 400°F.

Place the marrowbones on a baking tray and season with salt. Roast for 15 minutes, until bones are golden brown and the marrow is cooked through.

Meanwhile, place the broth in a saucepan and bring to a simmer over medium heat. Add the onion and simmer for 5 minutes, until the onion is tender. Add the Swiss and rainbow chard and cook for 5 to 8 minutes, until they are softened. Season with salt and pepper.

Scoop the marrow from the roasted bones and add to the broth, then gently stir in the lemon juice to taste.

Ladle the broth into bowls and serve, if you like a little heat, with some chili flakes sprinkled on top.

TIP: If rainbow chard is unavailable, you can use kale, but discard the tough stems.

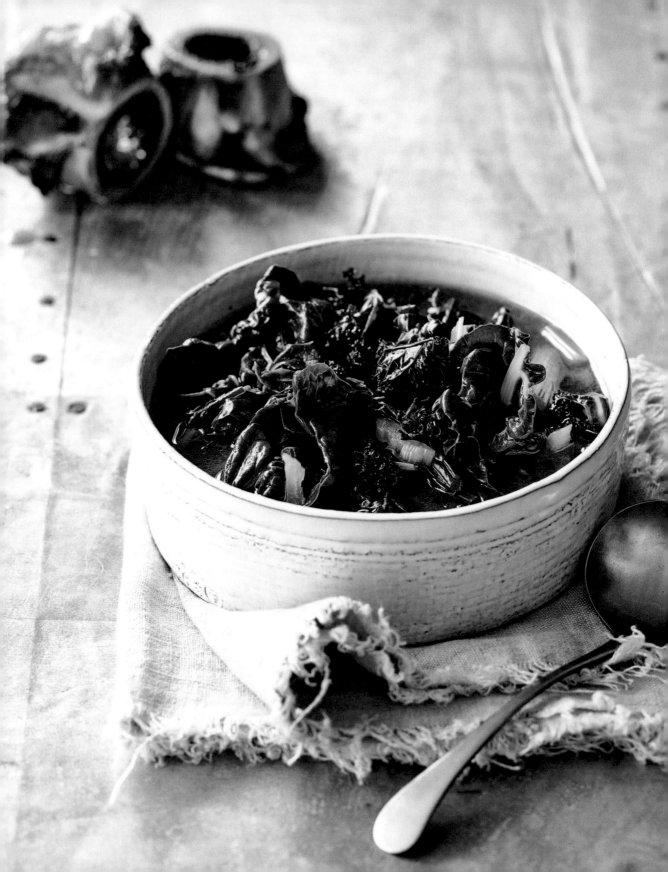

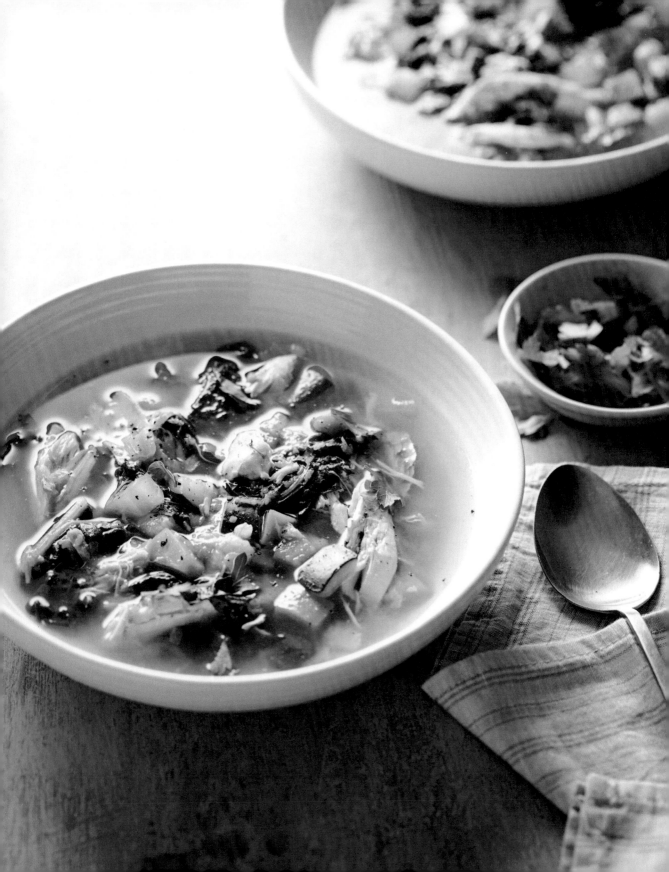

CHICKEN AND VEGETABLE COMFORT SOUP

It is said that the phrase "Winner, winner, chicken dinner" originates from 1970s casinos that were trying to attract players to underused tables. At the time, the most common bet was $2. Coincidentally, most casinos offered a chicken dinner for just under $2. Dealers would call out "Winner, winner, chicken dinner" when someone won the equivalent. How funny, then, that this dish costs about $2 per person and is one of the healthiest dishes in the world.

Heat the oil in a stockpot over medium heat. Add the onion, garlic, carrot, celery, thyme, and bay leaf. Cook, stirring occasionally, for 6 minutes, until the vegetables are soft but not browned.

Pour the broth into the pot and bring to a boil, then reduce the heat to low and simmer for 20 minutes.

Add the ginger, zucchini, and squash to the pot and cook for another 15 minutes, until the squash is tender. Add the chicken and chard and simmer for another few minutes until the chard is cooked.

Season the soup with salt and pepper and sprinkle with parsley before serving.

Serves: 6 to 8

2 Tbsp coconut oil or good-quality animal fat

1 onion, chopped

3 garlic cloves, finely chopped

1 large carrot, roughly chopped

1 celery stalk, halved lengthwise and cut into ½-inch slices

4 thyme sprigs

1 bay leaf

7 cups Chicken Bone Broth, plus extra if needed (see recipe, page 87)

1 Tbsp finely grated fresh ginger

1 zucchini, seeded, peeled, and cut into ¾-inch cubes

1 lb kabocha squash, cut into ¾-inch cubes

1 lb shredded poached chicken

½ lb Swiss chard, shredded

Sea salt and freshly ground black pepper

1 handful flat-leaf parsley leaves, finely chopped

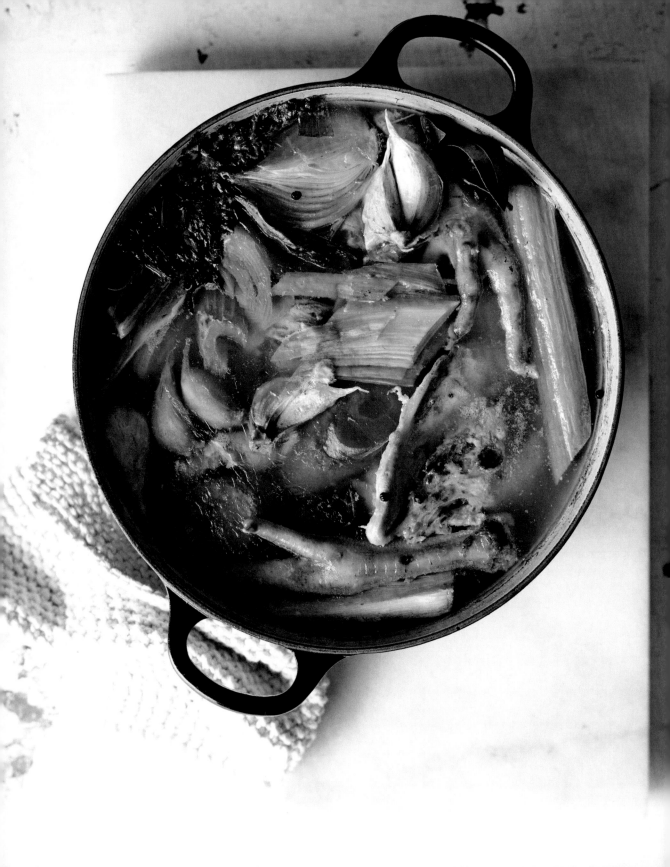

CHICKEN BONE BROTH

Place the chicken parts and the chicken feet, if using, in a stockpot or large saucepan. Add 5¼ quarts (21 cups) of cold water, the vinegar, onion, carrots, celery, leeks, garlic, parsley, and peppercorns and leave to stand for 30 minutes to 1 hour.

Bring to a boil, continuously skimming off the skin and foam that forms on the surface of the liquid. Reduce the heat to low and simmer for 6 to 12 hours. The longer you cook the broth, the more the flavors will develop.

Allow to cool slightly, then strain the broth through a fine sieve into a large storage container.

Cover and place in the refrigerator until the fat rises to the top and congeals. Skim the fat, and store both fat and broth in covered containers in your refrigerator or freezer. The reserved fat can be used as a cooking oil for meat, poultry, and vegetables dishes.

The broth can be stored in the refrigerator for up to 4 days or frozen for up to 3 months.

Makes: 1 gallon (16 cups)

3¼ lb bony chicken parts (necks, backs, breastbones, and wings)

2 to 4 chicken feet (optional)

2 Tbsp apple cider vinegar

1 large onion, roughly chopped

2 carrots, roughly chopped

3 celery stalks, roughly chopped

2 leeks (white part only), rinsed and roughly chopped

1 whole garlic bulb, cut in half crosswise

2 large handfuls flat-leaf parsley

1 Tbsp black peppercorns, lightly crushed

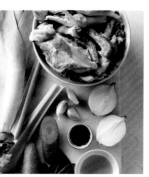 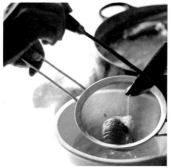 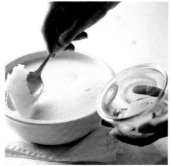 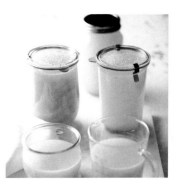

CHICKEN SOUP WITH AROMATIC SPICES

An oldie but a goodie, the classic chicken noodle soup cannot be beaten . . . unless you replace the gluten-containing, carb-loaded noodles with vegetable noodles to make it win-win for everyone. The flavor is better, your health will ultimately be better, and you are getting the nourishing goodness of a wonderful broth that has gelatin, collagen, calcium, glucosamine, magnesium, and a host of other benefits just waiting to be slurped up by the whole family. Be sure to make a huge batch so you can pack some in a thermos for a beautiful hot lunch.

Serves: 4

8 cups Chicken Bone Broth (see recipe, page 87)

2 lemongrass stems, pale part only, thinly sliced

2 cinnamon sticks

2 Tbsp finely grated ginger

4 chicken thighs, skin on

1 Tbsp coconut oil or good-quality animal fat

4 red Asian shallots, sliced

½ tsp ground turmeric

3 garlic cloves, sliced

1 spring onion, sliced

8 shiitake mushrooms, sliced

2 choy sum, trimmed and leaves separated

4 hard-boiled eggs, halved, to serve

Place the broth in a saucepan and bring to a boil. Add the lemongrass, cinnamon, ginger, and chicken. Bring back to a boil, reduce the heat to medium-low, and simmer for 5 minutes. Turn off the heat, cover with a lid, and leave the chicken to poach for 40 minutes, or until the juices run clear when the thickest part of the chicken is pierced with a knife. Carefully remove the chicken from the broth and, when cool enough to handle, remove and discard the bones. Set the broth and chicken aside, keeping warm. Skim any oil that rises to the top of the broth and reserve for cooking.

Meanwhile, to make the spice mix, toast the chili, peppercorns, coriander seeds, and cumin seeds in a saucepan until fragrant, 15 to 20 seconds. Remove from the heat and allow to cool. Finely grind the spices using a mortar and pestle or a spice grinder. Transfer to a small bowl, then mix in the salt. Set aside.

Heat the oil in a frying pan over medium heat. Add the shallots and cook for 5 minutes, until softened. Add the turmeric, garlic, spring onion, and shiitake and sauté for 2 minutes, until softened.

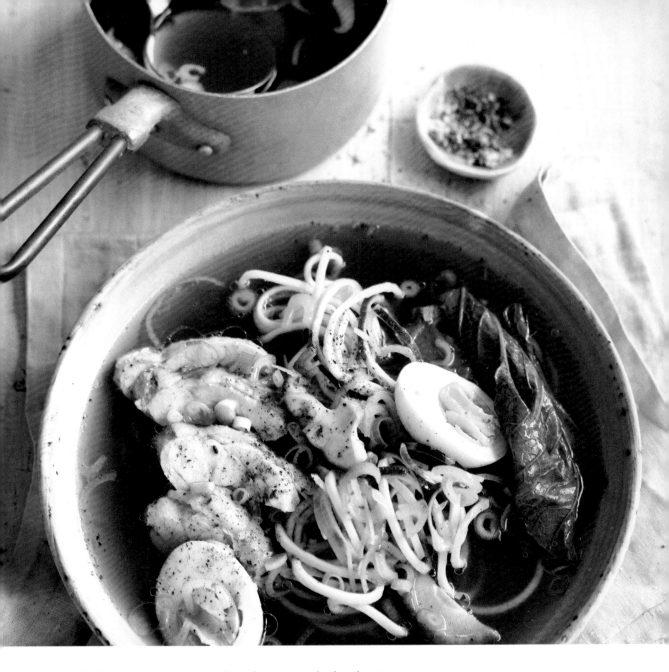

Add the sautéed shallots and mushrooms to the broth, stir in 1 tablespoon of the spice mix, and bring to a simmer. Add the choy sum and simmer for 3 minutes, until tender. Season with salt, if needed.

To serve, slice the chicken and arrange in a bowl, then add the choy sum and ladle the hot broth over the top. To finish, add two egg halves to each bowl and sprinkle on the remaining spice mix.

SPICE MIX

1 small dried chili

1 tsp black peppercorns

½ tsp coriander seeds

½ tsp cumin seeds

2 tsp sea salt

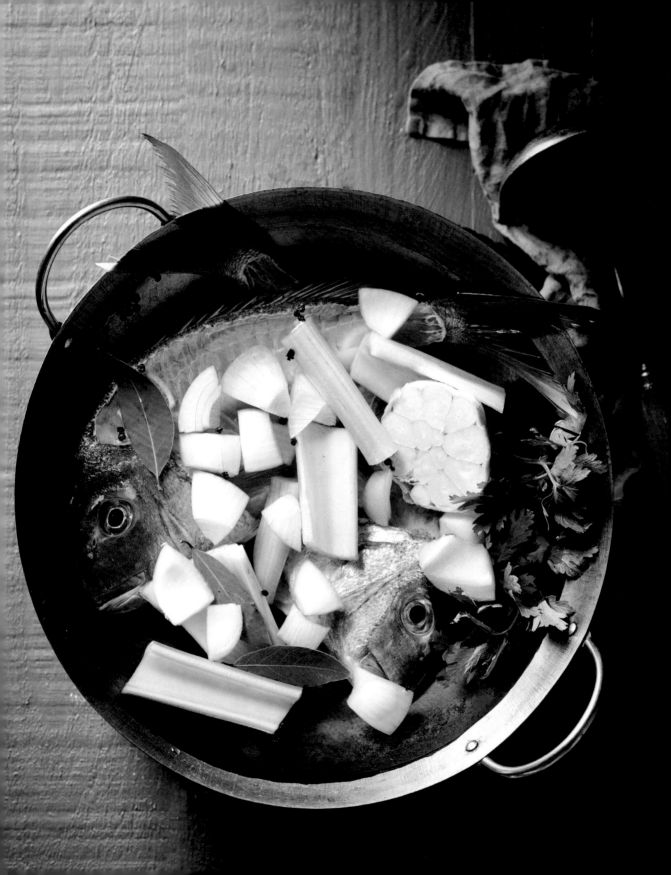

FISH BONE BROTH

Whenever you have a whole fish, make sure you keep the head and bones so you can make a delicious broth. Fish bone broth can be used as an aromatic base to create the most amazing soups and curries. All you need to do is add seafood, vegetables, spices, and herbs, and voilà: you have dinner in mere minutes.

Place the fish carcasses and heads in a stockpot or very large saucepan. Add the celery, onions, carrot, and apple cider vinegar and cover with 4 quarts of cold water.

Bring to a boil, skimming off the foam and any impurities as they rise to the top. Tie the thyme, parsley, and bay leaves together with kitchen string and add to the broth.

Reduce the heat to low, cover, and simmer for 3 to 4 hours until the broth is flavorsome and deepens in color.

Remove the fish carcasses and heads with tongs or a slotted spoon. Strain the broth into storage containers, cover, and chill in the refrigerator. Remove the congealed fat that rises to the top, if desired. It can be stored in a glass container in the fridge for up to 2 weeks and used for frying and sautéing. The broth can be stored in the refrigerator for up to 4 days or frozen for up to 3 months.

Makes: About 3 quarts

3 or 4 carcasses and heads of non-oily fish

2 celery stalks, roughly chopped

2 onions, roughly chopped

1 carrot, roughly chopped

2 Tbsp apple cider vinegar

1 handful of thyme and flat-leaf parsley sprigs

3 fresh or dried bay leaves

FRENCH ONION SOUP

How can anyone say no to a French onion soup that is so full of delicious, gut-healing beef broth, health-giving onion (known for regulating blood sugar), and medicinal garlic and thyme? Enjoy this when you want a nourishing breakfast, lunch, or dinner. If you want a heartier dish, add some bone marrow, braised short ribs, or beef marrow.

Serves: 4 to 6

2 Tbsp coconut oil or good-quality animal fat

3 lb onions, sliced

4 garlic cloves, chopped

2 tsp finely chopped thyme leaves

6 cups Beef Bone Broth, Chicken Bone Broth (see recipes, pages 77 and 87), or vegetable stock

2 bay leaves

Sea salt and freshly ground black pepper

2 macadamia nuts, activated if possible (i.e., soaked 4 to 8 hours in salted water), finely grated, to serve

Melt the oil in a large, heavy-based saucepan over medium-high heat. Add the onions and cook, stirring occasionally, for 30 minutes, until the onion is soft and beginning to brown.

Add the garlic and thyme, reduce the heat to medium-low, and cook, stirring occasionally, for 30 minutes, until the onion is caramelized.

Increase the heat to medium and, stirring constantly, gradually pour in the broth or stock. Then add the bay leaves.

Bring to a boil, skimming off any foam that rises to the surface. Reduce the heat to low and simmer gently for 50 minutes, until the soup is full of flavor with a nicely balanced sweetness. Season with salt and pepper.

Ladle the soup into bowls, sprinkle some grated macadamia over the top, and serve with paleo bread on the side.

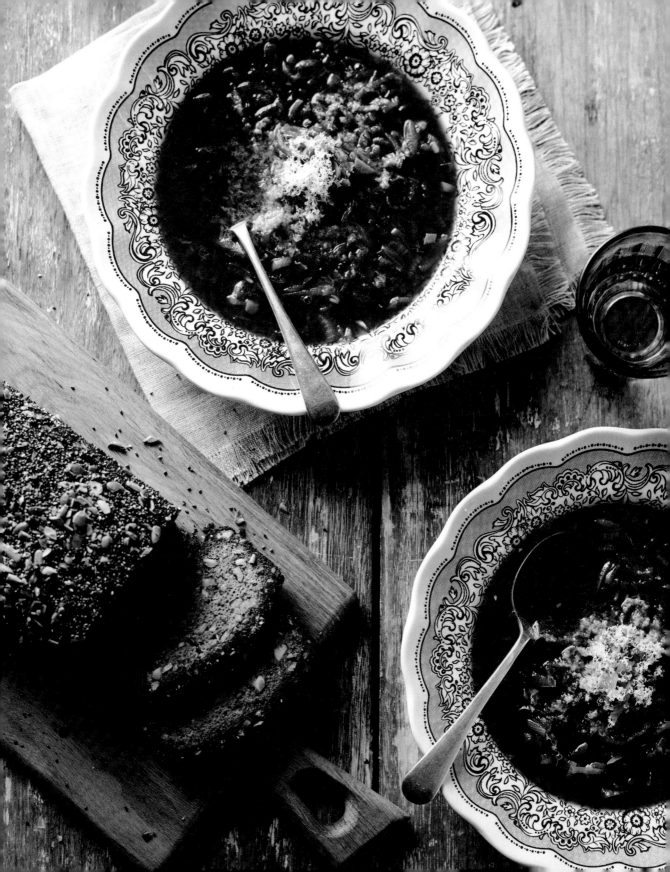

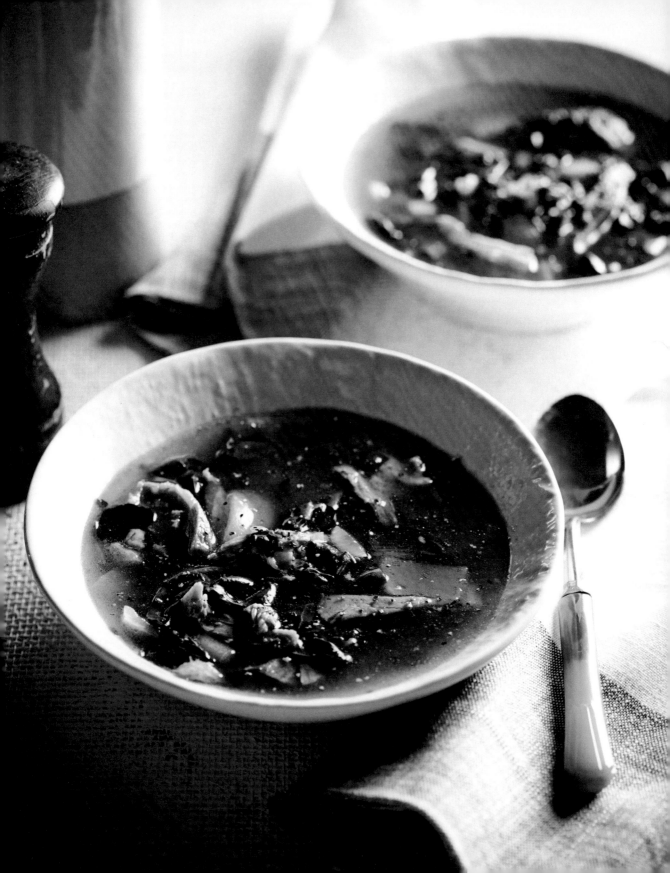

HEALING
HAM HOCK SOUP

We absolutely love soups, stocks, and broths. They are honestly food for the soul. Here, pasture-raised pork in the form of ham is a flavorful source of protein, and the inclusion of turmeric takes this dish to the next level. Turmeric, a bright yellow spice, has long been used in Chinese and Indian systems of medicine as an anti-inflammatory agent to treat a wide variety of conditions.

Heat the oil in a stockpot or very large saucepan over medium heat. Add the onions and cook, stirring often, for 3 to 5 minutes, until soft. Add the ham hock, garlic, celery, carrots, and turnip. Pour in the stock or water, stir in the turmeric and cumin, and bring to a boil. Reduce the heat to low, cover, and simmer for 1½ to 2 hours, until the meat is just starting to fall off the bone. The ham hock must be completely submerged during cooking, so add a little more stock or water if necessary.

Add the zucchini and pumpkin to the pot and cook for another 30 minutes, or until the zucchini and pumpkin are soft and the meat is falling off the bone.

Remove the ham hock from the soup, and once it is cool enough to handle, remove the meat from the bone, discarding the skin and fat. Shred or chop the meat and return to the pot. Stir in the chard and cook 5 minutes, until heated through. Stir in the lemon juice and season with salt and pepper.

Ladle the soup into warm bowls and serve.

Serves: 6

1 Tbsp coconut oil or other good-quality fat

2 onions, chopped

1 large smoked ham hock (about 2 to 2½ lb)

3 garlic cloves, sliced

2 celery stalks, sliced

2 carrots, peeled and thinly sliced

1 turnip, cut into ½-inch cubes

3 quarts chicken stock or water

1½ tsp ground turmeric

½ tsp ground cumin

2 zucchini, seeded, peeled, and cut into ½-inch cubes

¾ lb pumpkin, cut into ¾-inch pieces

2 large handfuls of Swiss chard leaves, stalks removed, roughly chopped

Juice of 1 lemon

Sea salt and freshly ground black pepper

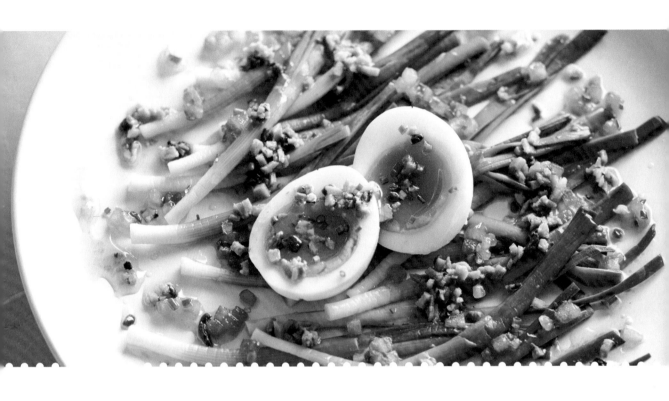

BREAKFAST

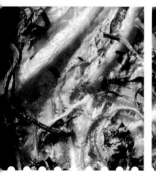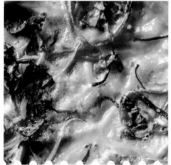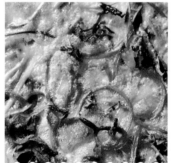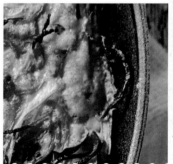

COCONUT YOGURT POTS
WITH FRESH BERRIES

Coconut yogurt is pretty perfect: it's low in carbs and high in fat, plus it contains some wonderful probiotic goodness. Add to that the delicious, creamy taste and it gets a double thumbs-up from Pete. This recipe is super easy to make, and you can flavor it with any spices you like, such as vanilla, cinnamon, or ginger.

Serves: 4

1 Tbsp powdered gelatin

5 cups coconut cream

Seeds of 1 split vanilla pod (optional)

1 to 2 Tbsp honey, maple syrup, or coconut sugar

4 capsules of Dr. Mercola Complete Probiotics or 1 packet of Kinetic Culture for Yogurt

1 Tbsp lemon juice (optional)

You'll need a 1½-quart preserving jar with a lid for this recipe. Wash the jar and all utensils thoroughly in very hot water or run them through a hot rinse cycle in the dishwasher.

Place 3 tablespoons of filtered water in a small bowl, sprinkle on the gelatin, and soak for 2 minutes.

Place the coconut cream and vanilla seeds (if using) in a saucepan and gently heat, stirring with a spoon, over medium-low heat until just starting to simmer (200°F, if testing with a thermometer). Do not allow to boil. Immediately remove the pan from the heat. While still hot, stir in the gelatin mixture, then add the honey and mix well. Cover the pan with a lid and set aside to cool to lukewarm (100°F or less).

Pour ½ cup of the cooled coconut milk mixture into a sterilized bowl. Open the probiotic capsules (if using). Stir the probiotic powder or starter culture and lemon juice (if using) into the coconut milk in the bowl. Add the remaining coconut milk and mix well.

Pour the coconut milk mixture into the sterilized jar and loosely seal the lid. Ferment in a warm spot for 12 hours at 100 to 105°F. To maintain this temperature and allow the yogurt to culture, wrap your jar in a tea towel and place it on a plate in the oven with the door shut and the oven light on. The light's warmth will keep the temperature

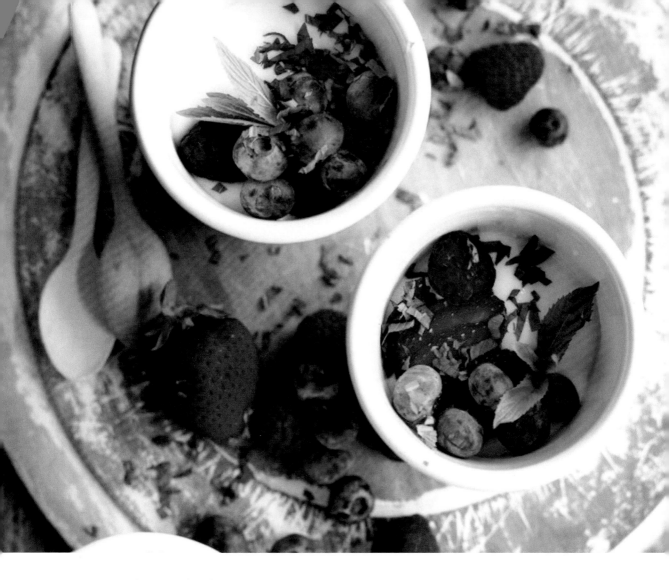

consistent. Alternatively, place the tea towel–wrapped jar in a cooler, fill a heatproof container with boiling water, and place it beside the jar without allowing them to touch. Close the lid. Replace the boiling water halfway through the fermenting process.

Once fermented, the yogurt will probably have air bubbles and look as though it has separated. Stir the fermented yogurt well and refrigerate for at least 5 hours before eating. If it separates after chilling, give it a good whisk. Store it in the fridge for up to 2 weeks.

To serve, divide the yogurt among four ramekins, cups, or serving bowls. Top with the fresh berries and garnish with mint.

TO SERVE:

1 cup fresh blueberries

½ cup fresh strawberries

½ cup fresh raspberries

Fresh mint leaves, some finely chopped and some left whole

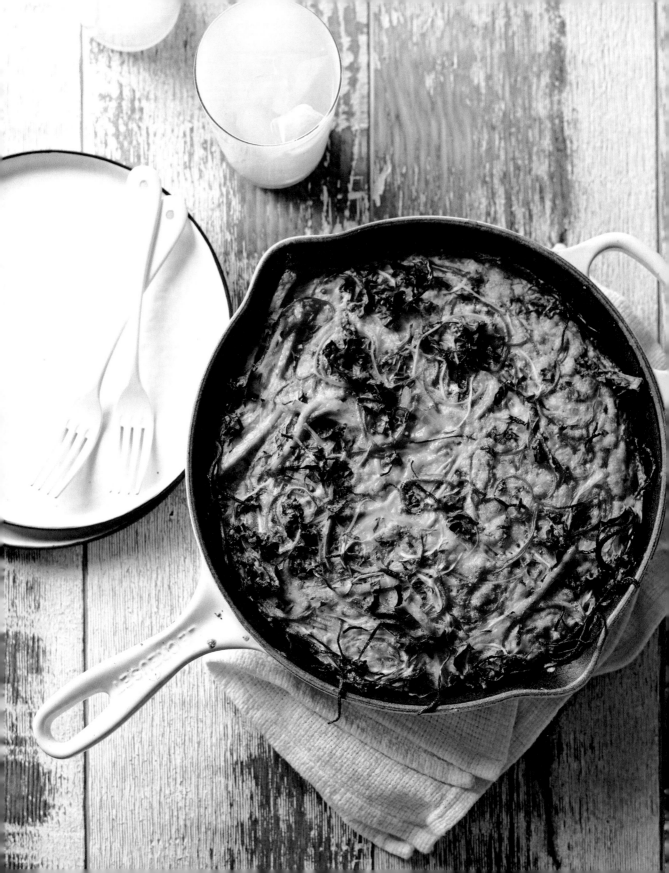

FRITTATA WITH LOADS OF VEGGIES

If there is one saving grace for busy, hungry families, it has to be the classic frittata. It is great for school or work lunches and perfect for when hungry teenagers ask what there is to eat, but the best part is that you can put basically anything in it and it tastes brilliant.

Last night's leftover roast beef, lamb, or chicken? Check! Things you need to use up in the fridge? Check! Vegetables to get into the kids' diets? Check! Give this frittata a whirl and make a big dish so you always have some on hand. Drizzle some homemade chili oil on top if you like it spicy.

Preheat oven to 400°F.

Combine the carrot, zucchini, and squash noodles in a bowl and set aside.

Crack the eggs into a bowl, add the parsley and coconut milk, and whisk lightly. Season well with salt and pepper and set aside.

Melt the oil in a large, ovenproof frying pan over medium heat. Add the onion and garlic and cook for 3 to 5 minutes, until soft. Stir in the bacon and cook for another 3 to 5 minutes, until light golden. Season with salt and pepper, add the noodles and spinach, and spread out evenly in the frying pan, then pour the egg mixture over the top. Transfer the pan to the oven and bake for 20 minutes, until the frittata is puffed and golden and cooked through.

Leave the frittata to cool for at least 10 minutes, then cut into portions in the pan or turn out onto a cutting board, cut into portions, and serve.

Serves: 6

1 carrot, spiral-cut into thin noodles

1 zucchini, seeded, peeled, and spiral-cut into thick noodles

½ lb kabocha squash or butternut squash, spiral-cut into thick noodles

8 eggs

2 Tbsp chopped flat-leaf parsley leaves

⅓ cup coconut milk

Sea salt and freshly ground black pepper

2 Tbsp coconut oil or good-quality animal fat

1 large onion, sliced

2 garlic cloves, crushed

7 oz rindless bacon or ham, chopped

1 large handful baby spinach or kale leaves

GREEN EGGS AND HAM

In honor of Dr. Seuss, one of Pete's daughters' favorites, we felt it would be great to reinterpret *Green Eggs and Ham* as a perfect school lunch or a picnic recipe that the whole family will enjoy.

Serves: 2

4 eggs

Melted coconut oil, for brushing

4 Tbsp finely chopped mixed herbs (such as flat-leaf parsley, thyme, basil, mint, and chervil)

4 to 6 slices of ham, to serve

Raw vegetables (lettuce, carrot and celery sticks, cherry tomatoes), to serve

Fill a small saucepan with water and bring to a boil over high heat.

Reduce the heat to low so that the water is simmering, then add the eggs and cook for 6 to 7 minutes. Drain and, when cool enough to handle, peel the eggs under cold running water.

Brush the peeled eggs with a little coconut oil, then roll the eggs in the herbs. Gently press in the herbs with the palm of your hands to create a nice, even coating.

Serve the green eggs with the ham and raw vegetables.

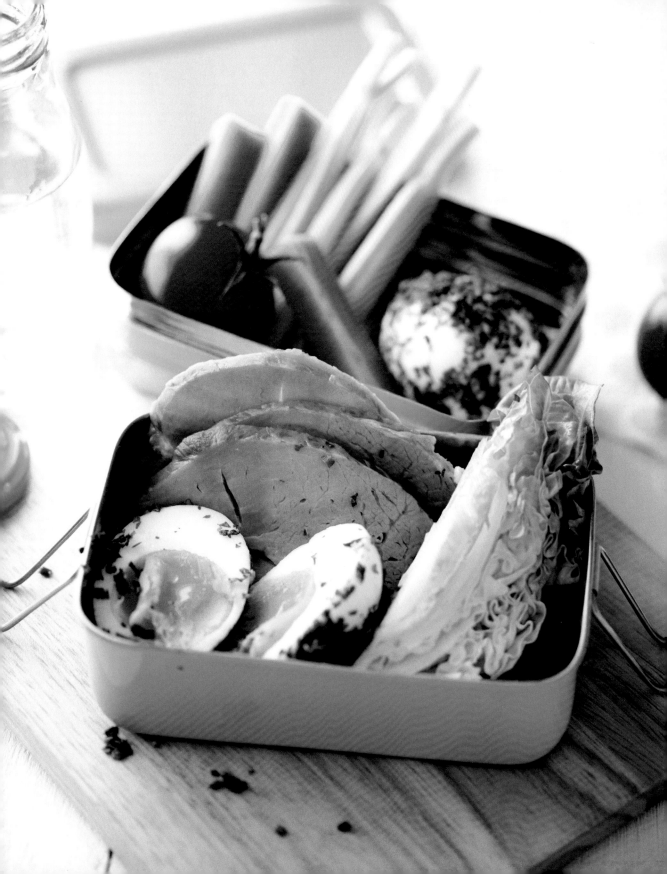

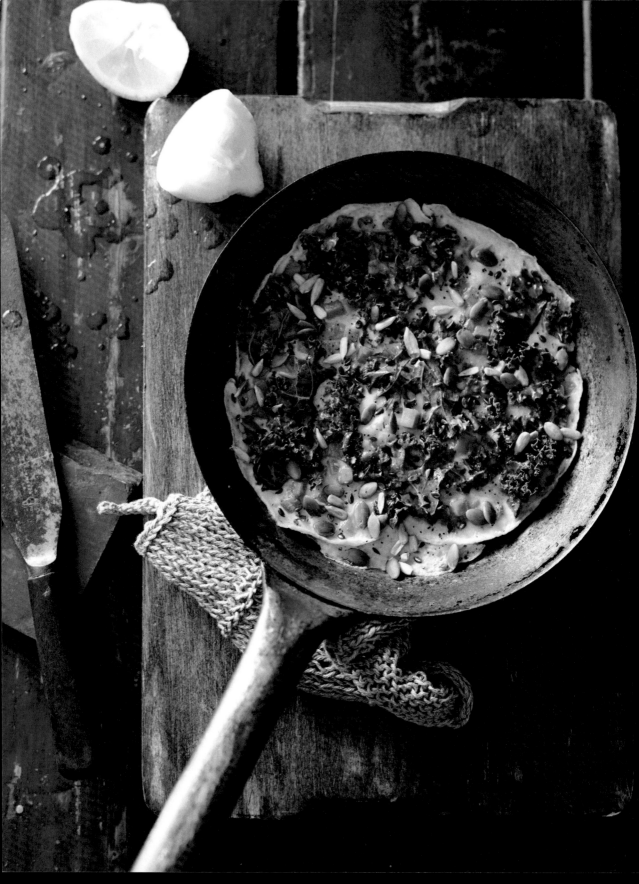

KALE AND PUMPKIN TORTILLA

This is a delicious and simple egg dish to make. It's the type of dish where any leftovers from the night before can be mixed and added to some eggs, then voilà: breakfast has never been so tasty or so quick—and there is no waste!

Leftovers are perfect to take to work or pack for the kids.

Wash the kale leaves thoroughly, then drain well and pat dry. Chop the kale roughly, place in a bowl (discard the inner stems), and set aside.

Break the eggs into another bowl and use a fork to lightly beat them. Season with salt and pepper.

Heat the coconut oil in a 9½-inch pan over medium heat. Add the pumpkin and cook for 3 minutes, then decrease the heat, add the garlic, and cook for 2 more minutes, or until softened. Increase the heat to medium, add the kale, and cook for 1 minute, stirring constantly.

Spread the kale and pumpkin into a single layer in the pan and pour the beaten eggs over the vegetables, swirling the egg mixture around the pan evenly. Reduce the heat to low and cook without stirring for 2 to 3 minutes, until almost cooked through. Remove the pan from the heat, cover with a lid and leave covered for 3 minutes to allow the residual heat in the pan to finish cooking the tortilla.

Cut the tortilla in half and gently slide each half off the pan onto two warm plates. Sprinkle with toasted pumpkin seeds and a light squeeze of lemon. Serve with a tablespoon of cultured vegetables of your choice on each plate.

Serves: 2

½ cup kale leaves

6 pastured organic eggs

Sea salt and freshly ground black pepper

2 Tbsp coconut oil or fat of your choice (e.g., duck fat, lard, or tallow)

½ cup pumpkin, peeled and cut into ¼-inch cubes

1 garlic clove, finely chopped

⅛ cup presoaked pumpkin seeds, toasted

Fresh lemon, to serve

2 Tbsp cultured vegetables or fermented kraut of your choice, to serve

MANU'S BABY LEEKS WITH SOFT-BOILED EGG, TRUFFLED BACON, AND SHERRY VINAIGRETTE

Pete's dear friend Manu Feildel is a classically trained French chef from Brittany on the French coast. French cuisine is one of Pete's favorites, and he asked Manu if he would share a salad. Manu told Pete about his leek salad with egg, bacon, and tomato, which sounded mighty good to him.

When we were photographing this recipe, we found the most gorgeous baby leeks, but if you can't find any, simply use larger leeks and cook them a little longer. Or, for a variation, replace the leeks with grilled asparagus. Thanks, Manu, and bon appétit!

Serves: 2 (as a starter)

15 baby leeks, trimmed and washed

2 Tbsp finely snipped chives

2 roma tomatoes, peeled, seeded, and finely diced

1 Tbsp extra-virgin olive oil

Sea salt and freshly ground black pepper

4 Tbsp Bacon and Sherry Vinaigrette (see recipe opposite)

1 Tbsp truffle oil (see note)

1 soft-boiled egg, peeled

Bring a saucepan of lightly salted water to a boil. Add the leeks and cook until tender, about 1 minute. Drain and refresh in ice-cold water. Drain again, shaking off any excess water, and pat dry with a paper towel.

Place the chives, tomatoes, and olive oil in a bowl, season with salt and pepper, and toss gently to combine. Set aside until needed.

Mix the Bacon and Sherry Vinaigrette with the truffle oil.

To serve, arrange the leeks on a serving platter or on two serving plates, scatter on the tomato and chive mixture, then slice the egg in half and pop on top. Drizzle with the truffled Bacon and Sherry Vinaigrette to finish.

NOTE: Truffle oil is an oil that has been infused with truffle, a fungus that grows underground. The oil has a strong mushroom-like flavor and is available at gourmet food stores and supermarkets.

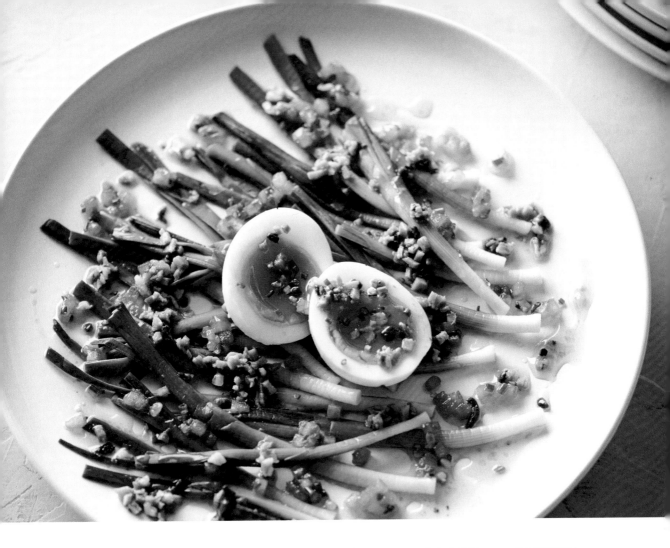

Heat half of the coconut oil in a small saucepan over low heat. Add the shallot and cook for 5 minutes, until soft. Remove from the pan.

Add the remaining coconut oil and the bacon to the pan and fry over medium heat, stirring occasionally, for 6 to 8 minutes, until the bacon is golden. Stir in the vinegar and shallot and set aside for about 5 minutes to cool.

Transfer the bacon and shallot mixture to a bowl and whisk in the mustard, chives, and olive oil. Season with salt and pepper. Store in a glass jar in the fridge for up to 1 week. Shake well before using.

BACON AND SHERRY VINAIGRETTE

Makes: About 1 cup

1 Tbsp coconut oil

½ French shallot, finely chopped

¼ lb rindless bacon, finely diced

4 Tbsp sherry vinegar or apple cider vinegar

1 tsp Dijon mustard

1 tsp finely snipped chives

½ cup extra-virgin olive oil

Sea salt and freshly ground black pepper

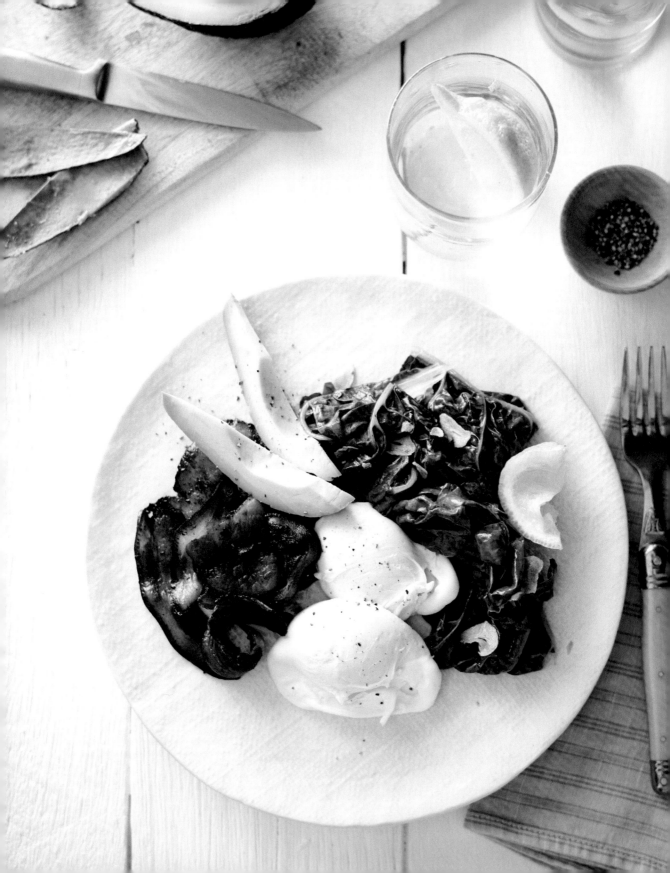

POACHED EGGS WITH BACON, AVOCADO, AND CHARD

To poach the eggs, pour the vinegar into a saucepan of boiling salted water, then reduce the heat to medium-low so the water is just simmering. Crack an egg into a cup. Using a wooden spoon, stir the simmering water in one direction to form a whirlpool and drop the egg into the center. Repeat with the remaining eggs and cook for 3 minutes, or until the eggs are done to your liking. Use a slotted spoon to remove the eggs, then place them on some paper towels to soak up the excess water.

Heat half of the oil in a nonstick frying pan over medium-high heat. Add the bacon and fry for 3 minutes on each side, until slightly colored (cook longer if you like it crisp). Remove from the pan, drain the excess oil on a paper towel, and keep warm.

To finish, heat a touch more oil in the pan, add the garlic, and cook until fragrant, about 20 seconds. Stir in the chard and cook until it is wilted, 1 to 2 minutes. Season with salt and pepper.

To serve, divide the chard among four warm serving plates, then top with two slices of bacon and a poached egg. Divide the avocado slices among the plates and sprinkle on some salt, pepper, and chopped parsley. Serve with cultured vegetables.

Serves: 4

2 Tbsp apple cider vinegar

4 free-range eggs

1 Tbsp coconut oil or other good-quality fat

8 slices free-range bacon

2 garlic cloves, thinly sliced

2 Swiss chard leaves, roughly chopped (reserve stalks for making bone broth)

Sea salt and freshly ground black pepper

1 avocado, sliced

1 Tbsp chopped flat-leaf parsley leaves, to serve

4 Tbsp cultured vegetables of your choice, to serve

SCRAMBLED EGGS WITH ROASTED BONE MARROW

This breakfast dish has delicious fat in the form of bone marrow (roasted in the oven), served with eggs, fermented veggies, and fresh herbs. If you don't have bone marrow, serve the eggs with avocado, bacon, or even a piece of grilled fish.

Serves: 2

1¼ lb center-cut beef marrowbones, cut into 1½-inch pieces, tendons trimmed (ask your butcher to do this)

4 eggs

2 Tbsp coconut cream or almond milk

2 Tbsp coconut oil or other good-quality fat, melted

Sea salt and freshly ground black pepper

4 chives, snipped into 1-inch lengths

Preheat the oven to 400°F.

Place the marrowbones on a baking tray and season with salt. Roast for 15 minutes, or until the bones are golden brown and the marrow is cooked through.

Meanwhile, using a fork, whisk the eggs, coconut cream, and 1 tablespoon of the oil in a bowl, then season with salt and pepper.

Heat the remaining oil in a nonstick frying pan over medium heat. Pour in the egg mixture and stir gently with a wooden spoon, lifting and pushing the egg mixture from the outside to the center until the eggs are almost set, about 2 minutes. Remove from heat, gently fold the mixture a few times, and leave to stand for 30 to 60 seconds, allowing the residual heat to finish cooking the eggs.

Divide the eggs between 2 serving plates and garnish with the chives, then add 2 or 3 pieces of roasted marrowbone sprinkled with pepper. Serve with fermented vegetables and watercress on the side.

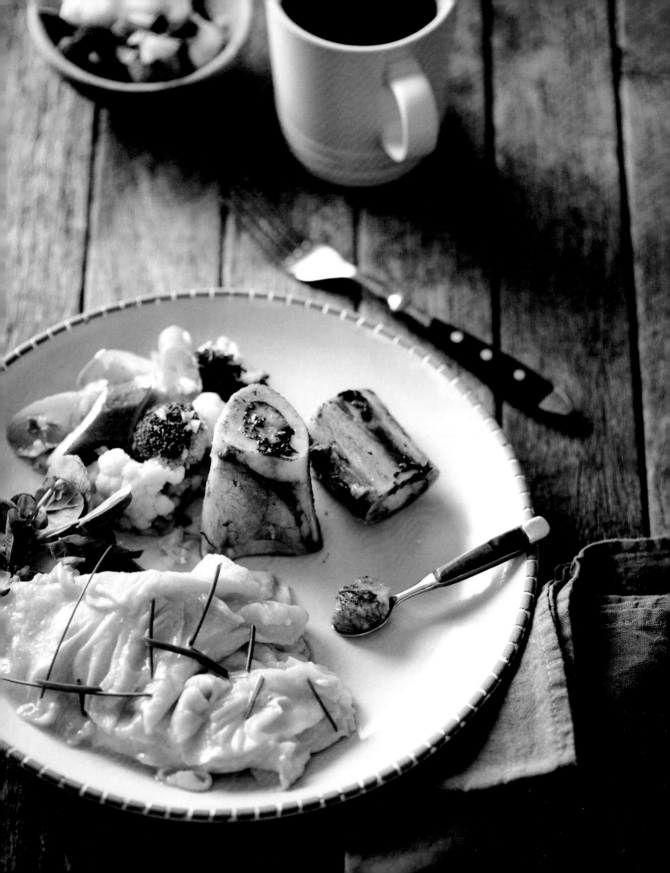

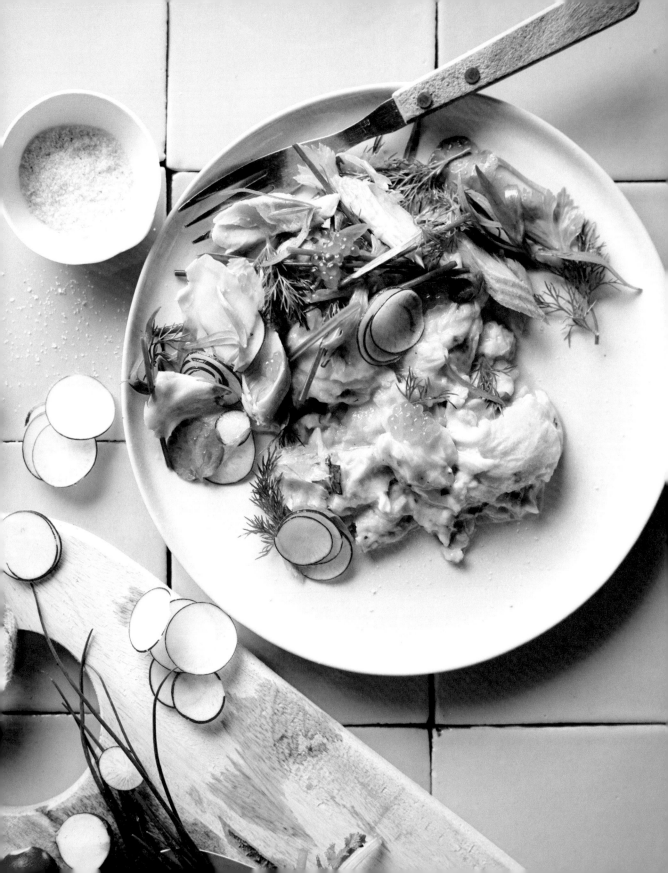

SCRAMBLED EGGS WITH SMOKED TROUT AND HERBS

These eggs are super easy and will take no more than 10 minutes to get from the fridge to your breakfast plate. Always spend your money on the best eggs you can find. Most free-range eggs are a far cry from what you might imagine; "free range" could just mean that the chickens have a piece of land for themselves that's about the size of an 8½-by-11 piece of paper, and the ground is dirt.

Look for pasture-raised, organic eggs to ensure that the chickens have the ability to peck for insects and to eat a balanced diet. This in turn produces the most nutritious eggs for us to consume. You can omit the fish from this dish, perhaps replacing it with some sautéed greens. Sprinkle on some roasted activated nuts, or even fold in some of last night's leftover Bolognese sauce.

Gently toss the radishes, artichokes, and herbs in a small bowl with the Mustard Vinaigrette. Whisk the eggs, coconut cream, and chives in a bowl and season with salt and pepper.

Melt the oil in a nonstick frying pan over medium heat, pour in the egg mixture, and stir gently with a wooden spoon for 2 to 3 minutes, until the eggs are set.

Divide the eggs between 2 plates and top with the trout and the herb salad. Serve with lemon wedges.

Serves: 2

3 radishes, thinly sliced

2 marinated artichoke hearts, flaked

2 handfuls of fresh mixed herbs (e.g., tarragon, chives, dill, flat-leaf parsley, watercress, celery leaves)

Mustard Vinaigrette (see recipe on next page)

4 eggs

2 Tbsp coconut cream

2 chives, finely chopped

Sea salt and freshly ground black pepper

1 Tbsp coconut oil or other good-quality fat

½ lb smoked trout, flaked

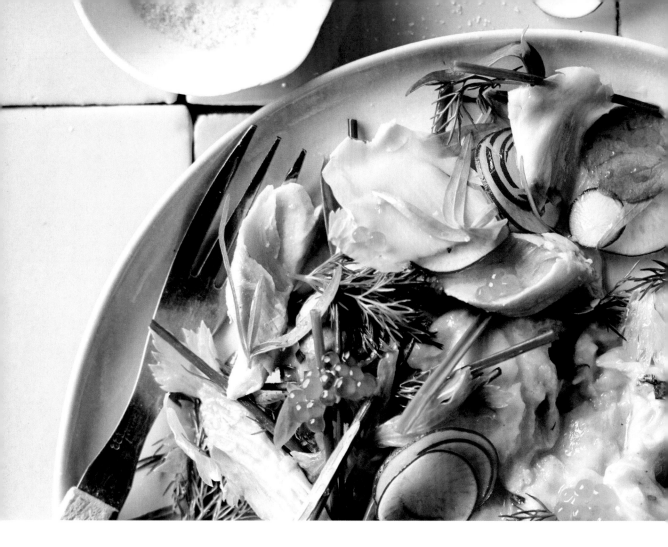

MUSTARD VINAIGRETTE

Makes: 1½ cups

4 Tbsp apple cider vinegar or lemon juice

2 Tbsp Fermented Mustard (see recipe opposite) or whole-grain mustard

1 tsp sea salt

¼ tsp freshly ground black pepper

1 garlic clove, crushed

1 cup extra-virgin olive oil or macadamia oil

Combine all the ingredients in a screw-top jar, cover, and shake well. Store in the refrigerator for up to 2 weeks. Shake well before using.

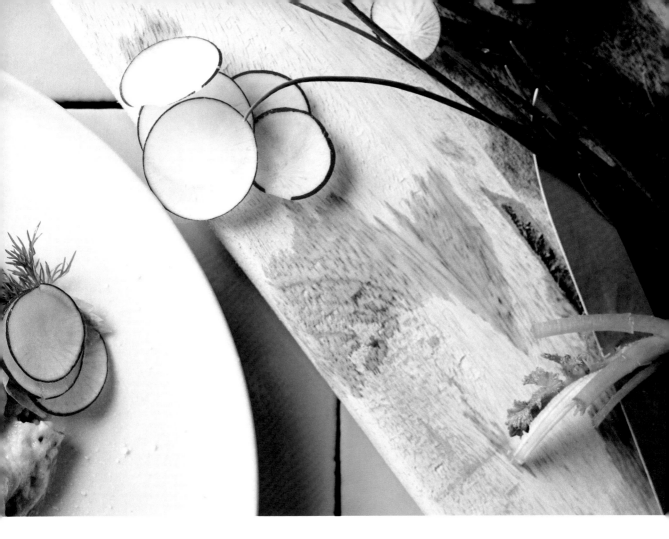

You will need a 250 ml (1 cup) preserving jar with an airlock lid for this recipe.

Wash the jar and utensils thoroughly in very hot water or run them through a hot rinse cycle in the dishwasher. Drain on a clean tea towel. Combine the fermented brine liquid, mustard seeds, shallot, and garlic in a glass or stainless steel bowl. Cover with a plate and allow to soak at room temperature overnight.

In a food processor, combine the soaked seed mixture with the maple syrup and process. If you like lots of whole seeds in your mustard, you will only need to process for a minute or two; if you like a smooth mustard, process for longer until you have a texture you are happy with. Check the seasoning and add sea salt to taste. Store in the preserving jar in the fridge, where it will keep for up to 3 months.

FERMENTED MUSTARD

Makes: About 1 cup

¾ cup fermented brine liquid, strained from one of the sauerkrauts

¾ cup brown and yellow mustard seeds (brown are hotter and will make a spicier mustard)

1 French shallot, finely chopped

2 garlic cloves, finely chopped

1 Tbsp maple syrup

Sea salt

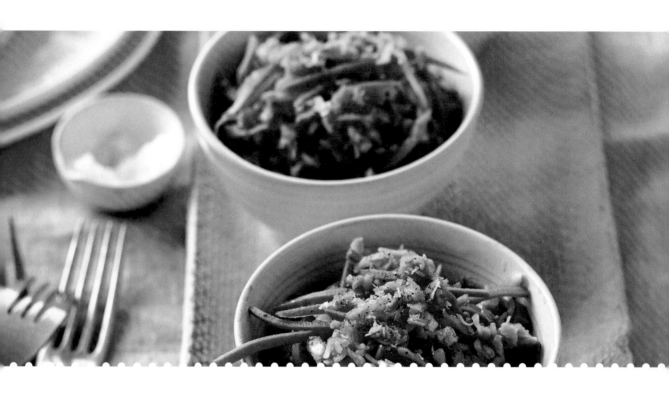

FERMENTED FOODS

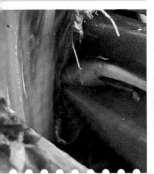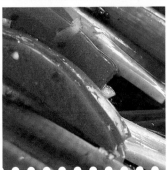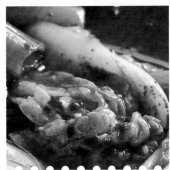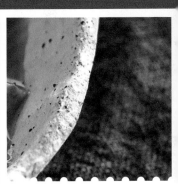

BEET KRAUT

Beet kraut goes with just about everything: roast beef, steak, all forms of pork—whether it be a roast with cracklings or bacon and eggs or slow-cooked ribs—as well as seafood (salmon in particular). It is also awesome on steak or in a salad. Give this a go once you have mastered the Beginner's Kraut (page 120).

Makes: 6½ cups

1 tsp black peppercorns

4 large beets, trimmed

¼ cabbage (green, red, or a mixture of the two)

Finely grated zest of 1 lemon

½ tsp toasted and ground wattle seeds (optional)

1½ tsp sea salt

½ packet starter culture, such as Dr. Mercola's Kinetic Culture Starter Kit for Vegetables

You will need a 1½-liter preserving jar with an airlock lid for this recipe. Wash the jar and all the utensils you will be using in very hot water or run them through a hot rinse cycle in the dishwasher.

Place the peppercorns in a small piece of muslin, tie it into a bundle, and set it aside. Shred the beets in a food processor or slice them into thin strips by hand or with a mandoline. Place the beets in a large glass or stainless steel bowl.

Remove the outer leaves of the cabbage. Choose one of the outer leaves, wash it well, and set it aside. Shred the cabbage in a food processor or slice it by hand or with a mandoline. Add the shredded cabbage, lemon zest, and wattle seeds (if using) to the beets, then add the salt. Mix well, cover, and set aside while you prepare the culture.

Dissolve the starter culture in filtered water according to the packet instructions (the amount of water will depend on the brand you are using). Add to the beet mixture along with the muslin bag containing the peppercorns and mix well.

Fill the prepared jar with the beet mixture, pressing down firmly with a large spoon or potato masher to remove any air pockets. Leave ¾ inch of room free at the top. The vegetables should be completely submerged in the liquid; add more water if necessary.

Take the clean cabbage leaf, fold it up, and place it on top of the beet mixture, then add a small sterile glass weight (a shot glass is ideal) to keep everything submerged. Close the lid, then wrap a tea towel around the jar to block out

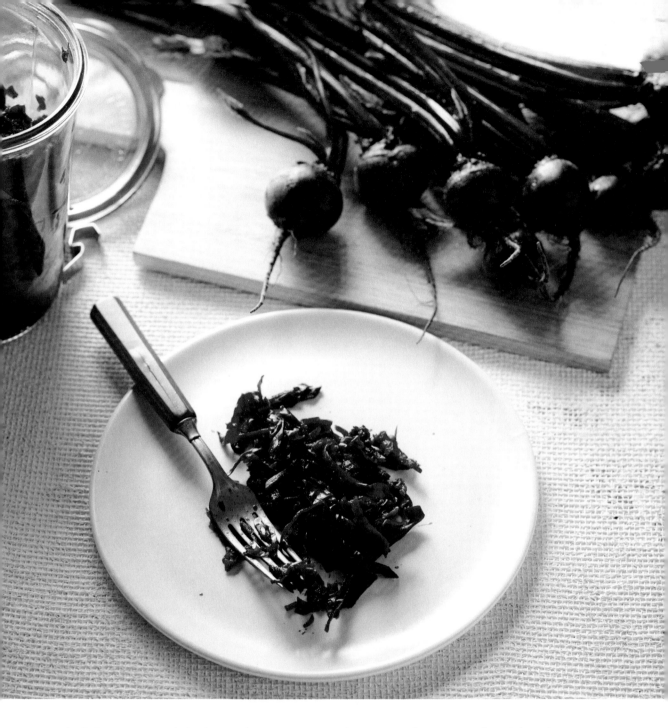

the light. Store in a dark place with a temperature of 50 to 75°F for 10 to 14 days. (Place the jar in a cooler to maintain a consistent temperature.) Different vegetables have different culturing times, and the warmer it is, the shorter the time needed. Remember to never heat fermented vegetables as this kills off their good bacteria. The longer you leave the jar, the higher the level of good bacteria and the more tangy the flavor.

BEGINNER'S KRAUT

Fermented vegetables will become a staple in homes over the next decade, not only because they taste amazing, but because of the scientific evidence coming out about how beneficial they are to our health. By including fermented vegetables in our diet, we are healing our second brain—our gut. The truth of the matter is that many diseases originate in the gut, so the goal is to make the gut super healthy. One of the ways we can do this is by encouraging healthy bacteria, and this child-friendly spice-free kraut is the perfect place to start. Try adding half a teaspoon per meal and gradually build up to 1 tablespoon per meal for children and perhaps 2 tablespoons for adults. This is super cheap to make, and you might even become addicted to it!

Makes: 1½ liters

1 lb green cabbage

1 lb red cabbage

1 beet, peeled

2 carrots, peeled (about ½ lb)

1½ tsp sea salt

1 packet starter culture, such as Dr. Mercola's Kinetic Culture Starter Kit for Vegetables

You will need a 1½-liter preserving jar with an airlock lid for this recipe. Wash the jar and all the utensils you will be using in very hot water. Alternatively, run them through a hot rinse cycle in the dishwasher. Remove the outer leaves of the cabbages. Choose an unblemished leaf, wash it well, and set it aside.

Shred the cabbages, beet, and carrots in a food processor or slice with a knife or mandoline, then transfer to a large glass or stainless steel bowl.

Sprinkle the salt over the vegetables, mix well, and cover with a plate. Prepare the starter culture according to the directions on the packet. Add to the vegetables and mix thoroughly.

Using a large spoon, fill the prepared jar with the vegetable mixture, pressing down firmly to remove any air pockets and leaving ¾ inch free at the top. The vegetables should be completely submerged in the liquid; add more water, if necessary.

Take the clean cabbage leaf, fold it up, and place it on top of the vegetables, then add a small glass weight (a sterile shot glass is ideal) to keep everything submerged. Close the lid and wrap a tea towel around the jar to block out the light. Store in a dark place with a temperature of 50 to 75°F for 10 to 14 days. (You can place the jar in a cooler to maintain a consistent temperature.)

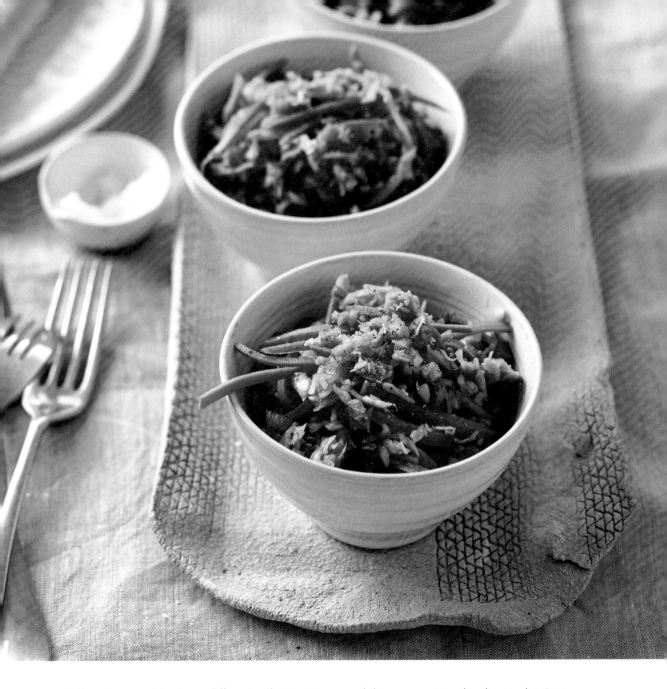

Different vegetables have different culturing times, and the warmer it is, the shorter the time needed. The longer you leave the jar, the higher the level of good bacteria present. It is up to you how long you leave it—some people prefer the tangy flavor that comes with extra fermenting time, while others prefer a milder flavor.

Chill before eating. Once opened, it will last for up to 2 months in the fridge when kept submerged in liquid. If unopened, it will keep for up to 9 months in the fridge.

CULTURED CARROTS

Fermenting the humble carrot might be the easiest way to introduce fermented vegetables to your family. We think nearly every kid on the planet loves carrots, so the positive association is already there. Now all you have to do is tell them that these are super carrots, and watch their eyes light up. You might want to get them to draw a cartoon character of a super carrot or make up a song about it. Remember: never heat fermented vegetables; this kills off the good bacteria. Serve them chilled or at room temperature. The fermented juice has so much goodness and can be combined with extra-virgin olive oil, herbs, and seasoning to make a delicious salad dressing.

Makes: 1½ liters

1 tsp black peppercorns

6 large carrots, peeled and thinly cut

1½ tsp sea salt

1 packet starter culture, such as Dr. Mercola's Kinetic Starter Kit for Vegetables

Zest of 1 orange, peeled off in long strips

2 cinnamon sticks

1 small cabbage leaf, washed

You will need a 1½-liter preserving jar with an airlock lid for this recipe. Thoroughly wash the jar and all the utensils you will be using in very hot water or run them through a hot rinse cycle in the dishwasher.

Place the peppercorns in a small piece of muslin, tie into a bundle with kitchen string, and set aside.

Place the carrots in a stainless steel bowl and sprinkle with salt. Mix well, cover, and set aside.

Dissolve the starter culture in water according to the packet instructions (the amount of water will depend on the brand you are using). Add to the carrots along with the muslin bag containing the peppercorns, the orange zest, and cinnamon sticks. Mix well.

Fill the prepared jar with the carrots, pressing down firmly with a large spoon to remove any air pockets and leaving ¾ inch of room at the top. The carrots should be completely submerged in the liquid, so add more water if necessary.

Take the clean cabbage leaf, fold it up, and place it on top of the carrots, then add a small glass weight (a sterile shot glass is ideal) to keep everything submerged. Close the lid, then wrap a tea towel around the jar to block out the light. Store in a dark place with a temperature of 50 to 75°F for 10 to 14 days. (You can place the jar in a cooler to maintain a consistent temperature.)

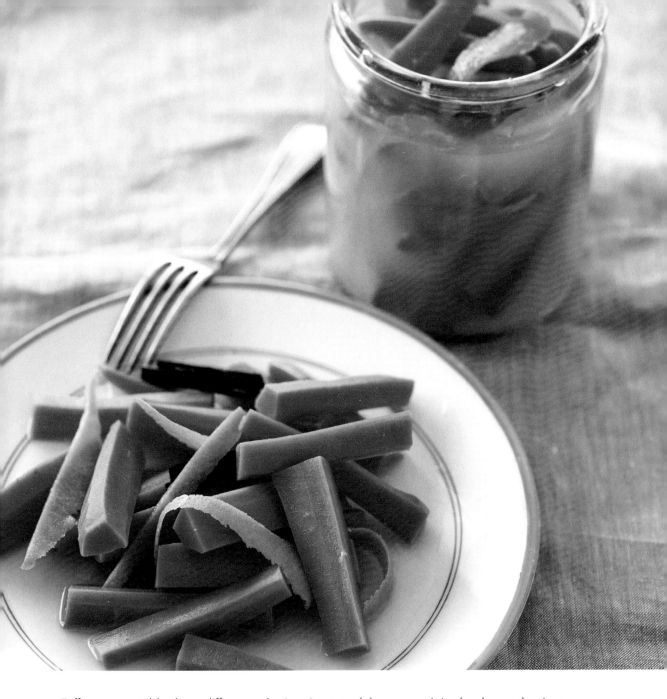

Different vegetables have different culturing times, and the warmer it is, the shorter the time needed. The longer you leave the jar, the higher the level of good bacteria present. It is up to you how long you leave it—some people prefer the tangy flavor that comes with extra fermenting time, while others prefer a milder flavor.

Chill before eating. Once opened, it will last for up to 2 months in the fridge when kept submerged in liquid. If unopened, it will keep for up to 9 months in the fridge.

KIMCHI

Kimchi is a Korean fermented cabbage condiment that will become a staple in your kitchen. Whenever we are cooking an Asian-inspired dish at home, such as eggs, curry, stir-fry, salad, or satay on the barbecue, out comes the kimchi to complement it. Play around with the spices, and if you don't like it hot, then simply reduce the amount of chili you use.

Makes: 1½ liters

1 Chinese cabbage (napa cabbage)

3 spring onions, thinly sliced

1½ tsp sea salt

3 garlic cloves, thinly sliced

2-inch piece fresh ginger, peeled, sliced, then julienned

2 to 3 Tbsp fish sauce

1 to 2 Tbsp Korean chili powder (gochugaru)

1 packet starter culture, such as Dr. Mercola's Kinetic Culture Starter Kit for Vegetables

You will need a 1½-liter preserving jar with an airlock lid for this recipe. Wash the jar and utensils thoroughly in very hot water or run them through a hot rinse cycle in the dishwasher.

Remove the outer leaves of the cabbage. Choose one, wash it well, and set it aside.

Cut the cabbage in half lengthwise, then crosswise into 2-inch pieces, discarding the root end.

Combine the cabbage with the spring onions. Add the salt and mix well. Add the garlic, ginger, fish sauce, and chili powder. Mix well, cover, and set aside.

Dissolve the starter culture in water according to the packet instructions (the amount of water will depend on the brand). Add to the vegetables and mix well. Fill the prepared jar with the vegetable mix, pressing down firmly between additions with a large spoon or potato masher to remove any air pockets. Leave ¾ inch of room free at the top. The vegetables should be completely submerged in the liquid, so add more water if necessary.

Fold the clean cabbage leaf, place it on top of the mixture, and add a small glass weight to keep everything submerged (a small sterile shot glass is ideal). Close the lid, then wrap a tea towel around the jar to block out the light. Store in a dark place with a temperature of 60 to 75°F for at least 10 days and up to 2 weeks. (You can place the jar in a cooler to maintain a consistent temperature.)

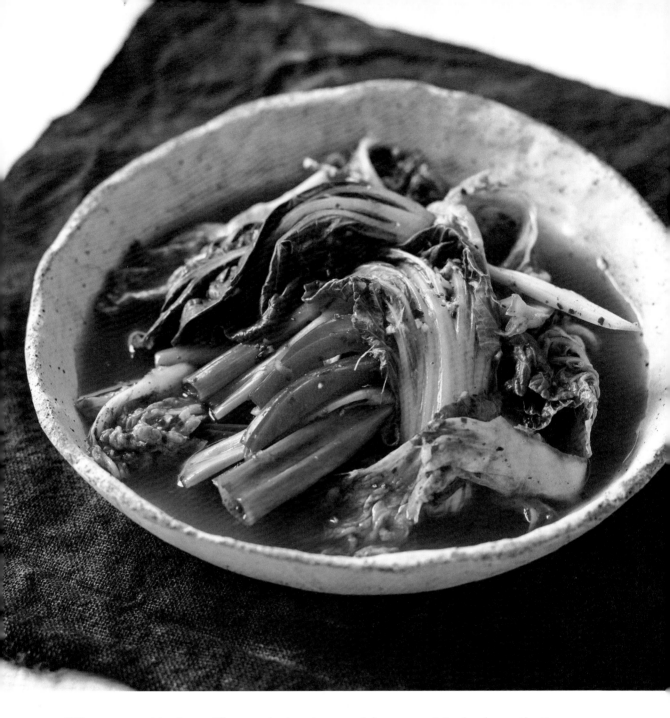

Different vegetables have different culturing times, and the warmer it is, the shorter the time needed. The longer you leave the jar to ferment, the more good bacteria will be present, and the more tangy the flavor.

Chill before eating. Once opened, the kimchi will last for up to 2 months in the fridge when kept submerged in the liquid. If unopened, it will keep for up to 9 months in the fridge.

SAUERKRAUT

In a perfect world, people would give jars of homemade sauerkraut as a gift for birthdays, Christmas, and Valentine's Day instead of boxes of sugar-laden chocolates! Real fermented sauerkraut (not the stuff on the supermarket shelf that isn't refrigerated) is the simplest and most effective way to create good gut health. On top of that, fermented veggies are cheap to make and absolutely delicious.

Makes: 6½ cups

1 star anise

1 tsp whole cloves

1¼ lb cabbage (green, red, or a mix of the two)

1½ tsp sea salt

2 tsp caraway seeds

2 Tbsp juniper berries

1 small handful dill, roughly chopped

1 packet starter culture, such as Dr. Mercola's Kinetic Culture Starter for Vegetables

You will need a 1½-liter preserving jar with an airlock lid for this recipe. Wash the jar and utensils thoroughly in very hot water or run them through a hot rinse cycle in the dishwasher.

Place the star anise and cloves in a small piece of muslin, tie into a bundle, and set aside. Remove the outer leaves of the cabbage. Choose one of the outer leaves, wash it well, and set it aside. Shred the cabbage in a food processor or slice by hand or with a mandoline, then place it in a large glass or stainless steel bowl.

Sprinkle the salt, caraway seeds, juniper berries, and dill over the cabbage. Mix well, cover, and set aside while you prepare the starter culture.

Dissolve the starter culture in water according to the packet instructions (the amount of water will depend on the brand you are using). Add to the cabbage along with the muslin bag containing the spices and mix well.

Fill the prepared jar with the cabbage mix, pressing down firmly between each addition with a large spoon or potato masher to remove any air pockets. Leave ¾ inch of room at the top. The cabbage should be completely submerged in liquid, so add more water if necessary.

Take the reserved cabbage leaf, fold it, and place it on top of the mixture, then add a small glass weight to keep everything submerged (a small sterile shot glass is ideal). Close the lid, then wrap a tea towel around the jar to block out the light. Store in a dark place with a temperature of 60 to 75°F

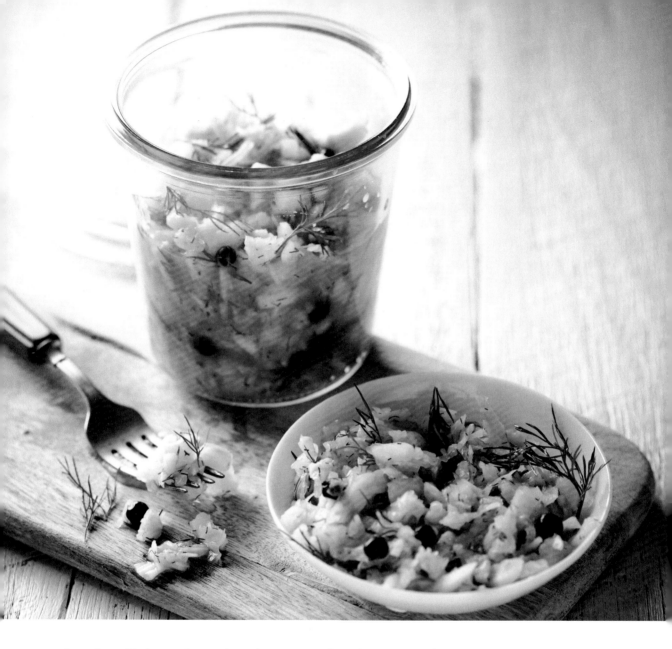

for at least 10 days and up to 2 weeks. (You can place the jar in a cooler to maintain a consistent temperature.)

Different vegetables have different culturing times, and the warmer it is, the shorter the time needed. The longer you leave the jar to ferment, the greater the level of good bacteria present. Some people prefer the tangy flavor that comes with extra fermenting time, while others prefer a milder flavor.

Chill before eating. Once opened, the sauerkraut will last for up to 2 months in the fridge when kept submerged in the liquid. If unopened, it will keep for up to 9 months in the fridge. As an added option, reserve some juice to make Beet Kvass (see recipe, page 201).

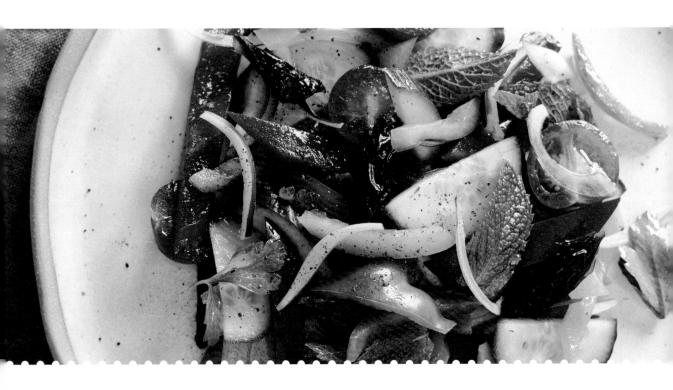

SALADS

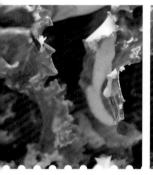
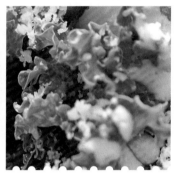
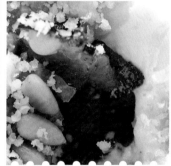
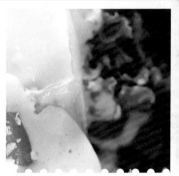

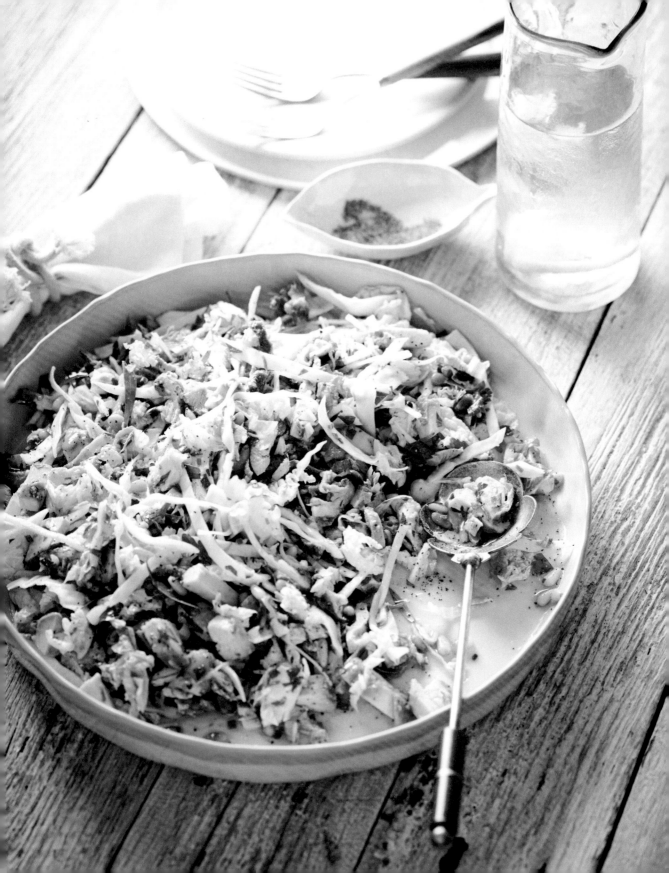

CREAMY CHICKEN AND CABBAGE SALAD

Cook up a couple of chickens during the week—you could roast them, strip the meat off, and make a broth from the bones, or you could poach them in a stock before stripping the meat off. In both cases you are left with a nutritious broth to drink on its own or add to soups, braises, or curries, as well as the chicken meat, which you can use to whip up a healthy meal.

This recipe comes from Pete's good friend naturopath Helen Padarin, and it's one of his favorite ways to use cooked chicken. You've got quality protein mixed with good fats and fibrous veggies, and you can have it on the table in less than 15 minutes. You can't argue with that!

Mash the avocado to a creamy and slightly chunky texture in a bowl, then add the cabbage, roast chicken, olive oil, and lemon juice and give everything a good toss so the avocado dresses the salad nicely. Season with salt and pepper.

Arrange the salad on a platter and sprinkle the pine nuts over the top.

Serves: 3 to 4

1 avocado, diced

½ medium-sized head savoy cabbage, shredded

1 cup roast chicken, shredded

3 Tbsp extra-virgin olive oil

3 Tbsp lemon juice

Sea salt and freshly ground black pepper

2 Tbsp pine nuts, soaked and toasted

CURLY ENDIVE
AND WALNUT SALAD

Curly endive contains good levels of vitamins A and K and folate. A bitter green leaf that has long been appreciated in Europe as a delicacy, it adds a wonderful texture and flavor to salads. You can also lightly cook it with some cinnamon and drizzle with olive oil and lemon juice, or add it to your favorite soups. If the flavor in this salad is a little overpowering for some members of the family, mix the endive leaves with less strongly flavored lettuces.

Serves: 4

½ curly endive, leaves separated and torn

2 to 3 roma tomatoes, cut into wedges

⅓ cup walnuts, activated if possible (i.e., soaked 4 to 8 hours in salted water), toasted and chopped

2 spring onions, green part cut into thin strips and soaked in cold water to curl, white part thinly sliced

2 Tbsp red wine vinegar or apple cider vinegar

½ tsp Dijon mustard

3 Tbsp extra-virgin olive oil

Sea salt and freshly ground black pepper

Place the endive, tomatoes, walnuts, and spring onions in a large salad bowl. Set aside.

To make the dressing, combine the vinegar, mustard, and olive oil in a small bowl, season with salt and pepper, and whisk well.

Pour the dressing over the salad and gently toss to coat. Season with more salt and pepper, if needed, and serve in a large salad bowl or on a platter.

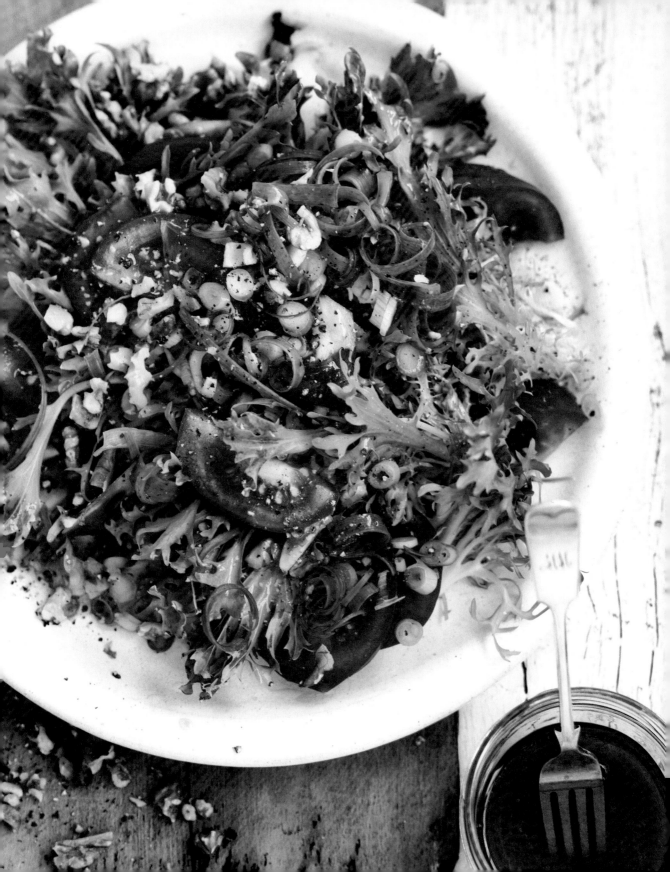

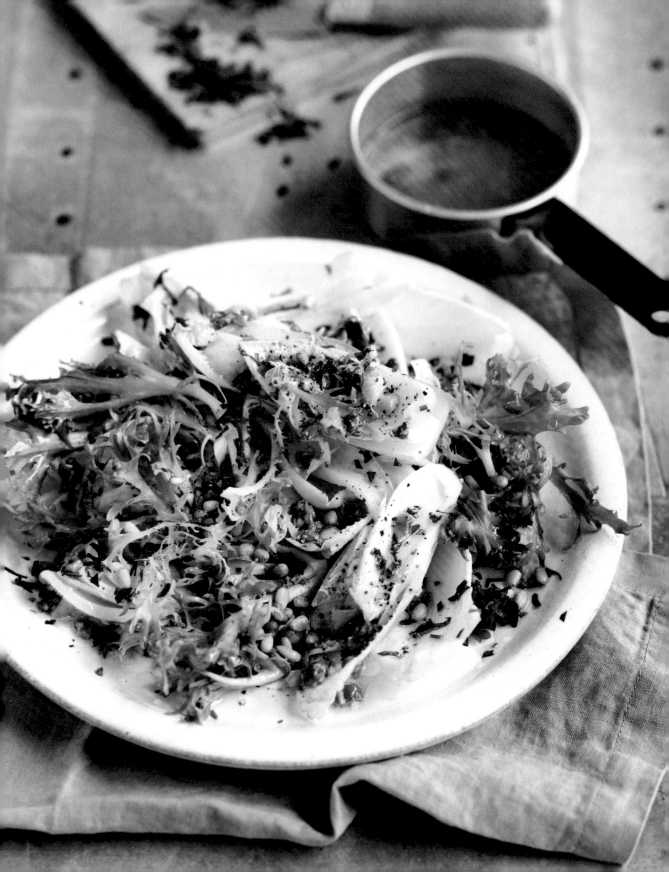

ENDIVE, PARSLEY, AND MACADAMIA NUT SALAD WITH ANCHOVY DRESSING

This easy-to-make salad of crisp and slightly bitter pale-green Belgian endive and curly endive leaves is so delicious with its anchovy dressing. You can also use this versatile dressing on grilled broccolini, lamb cutlets, or seafood.

To make the dressing, place all the ingredients in a bowl and mix to combine.

Arrange the Belgian endive and curly endive on a platter and pour the dressing over the leaves. Sprinkle on the macadamia nuts and parsley and serve.

Serves: 4

2 Belgian endive, trimmed and leaves separated

¼ head curly endive (about 4 ounces), leaves separated and roughly torn

1 oz macadamia nuts, slivered and toasted

3 Tbsp roughly chopped flat-leaf parsley

DRESSING

4 anchovy fillets, finely chopped

2 garlic cloves, finely grated

2 Tbsp apple cider vinegar

3 Tbsp extra-virgin olive oil

Sea salt and freshly ground black pepper

FENNEL, WATERCRESS, AND HERB SALAD WITH SHALLOT DRESSING

Pete is a huge lover of fennel and believes it is an underutilized vegetable. When it is in season he roasts, braises, and ferments it. This easy yet delicious fennel salad deserves a place on every dinner table. Simply serve it alongside some grilled fish or roasted meat.

Mint pairs perfectly with fennel and is a very good herb to start with, but feel free to play around with other herbs of your choice. You may also like to add some seeds or nuts such as walnuts, almonds, or macadamias for a bit of crunch.

Serves: 4

1 large fennel bulb, trimmed and shaved, fronds reserved

1 large handful watercress

1 handful mint leaves

1 handful dill fronds, shaved

SHALLOT DRESSING

1 French shallot, finely diced

3 Tbsp apple cider vinegar

1 tsp Dijon mustard

4 Tbsp extra-virgin olive oil

Sea salt and freshly ground black pepper

Using a mandoline or sharp knife, thinly shave the fennel.

Place the shaved fennel, watercress, mint, and dill fronds in a large bowl and set aside while you prepare the dressing.

To make the dressing, place all the ingredients in a small bowl and whisk to combine.

Pour only enough dressing over the salad to coat, then gently toss to combine. Check seasoning and add more salt and pepper if needed.

Arrange the fennel salad on a large platter and drizzle over a little more dressing, if desired.

TIP: Any leftover dressing can be stored in a sealed jar in the fridge for up to 2 weeks.

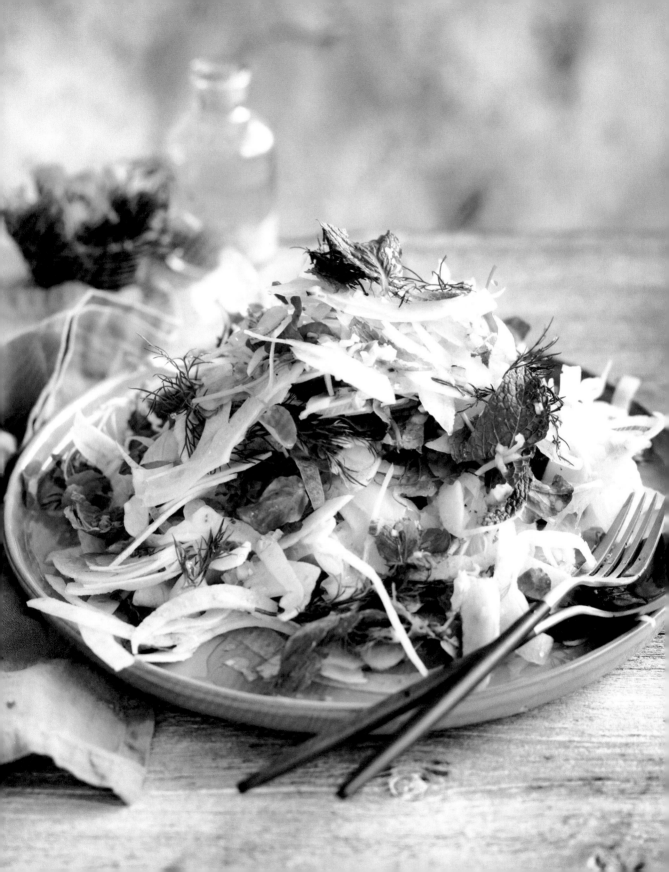

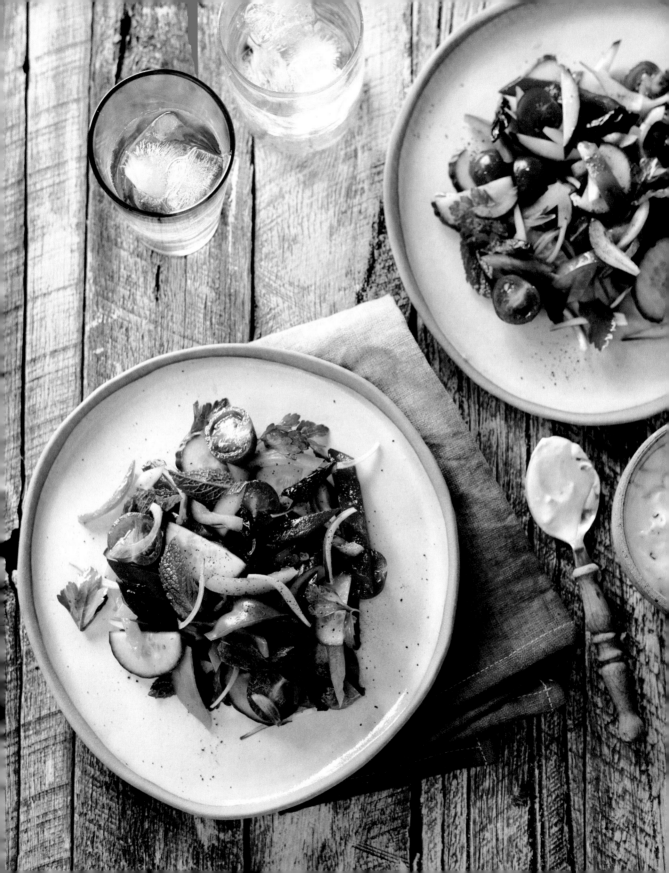

GYPSY SALAD

Pete adores salads like this one—salads that use top-quality spices, herbs, fruit, and vegetables; are put together in a matter of minutes; and just blow your taste buds away. His advice is to make a few delicious dressings and sauces throughout the week and keep them in the fridge to use in your salads; to accompany cooked meat, seafood, or vegetables; or to stir into your favorite soups. Play around with ingredients that are in season, and add a spoonful or two of fermented vegetables for gut health.

To make the coconut dressing, combine the garlic, chili, cumin, sumac, coconut yogurt, and lemon juice in a bowl, season with a little salt and pepper, and mix well.

To make the salad, place all the ingredients in a large bowl, season with salt and pepper, and gently toss to combine.

Place the salad on a serving dish and drizzle the coconut dressing on top. Sprinkle with some extra sumac to finish.

Serves: 4 as a side dish

1 cup cherry tomatoes, halved

1 peeled and seeded cucumber, halved lengthways and thinly sliced

½ red onion, finely sliced

5 medjool dates, pitted and sliced

½ yellow pepper, seeded and finely sliced

1 red pepper, seeded and finely sliced

½ green pepper, seeded and finely sliced

1 large handful mint leaves

1 large handful flat-leaf parsley leaves

Juice of ½ lemon

3 Tbsp extra-virgin olive oil

COCONUT DRESSING

1 garlic clove, finely chopped

1 small red chili, seeded and finely chopped

½ tsp ground cumin

½ tsp sumac, plus extra to serve

½ cup coconut yogurt

Juice of ½ lemon

Sea salt and freshly ground black pepper

ICEBERG WEDGE SALAD
WITH BACON AND EGG

Sometimes you just need a good iceberg salad to help you refresh, especially when it's hot outside. The fresh crispness of a cold iceberg lettuce is very hard to beat. It may not be the most nutritious of lettuces or leafy greens, but it makes for a welcome change. We love to add boiled eggs and bacon, smoked trout, or even leftover roast chicken, and then use a mayonnaise, tahini, or simple vinaigrette to dress it.

Serves: 6

1 tsp coconut oil or good-quality fat

4 rindless bacon rashers, cut into small dice

1 large iceberg lettuce, cored and cut into 6 wedges

4 hard-boiled eggs, chopped

½ cup Mayonnaise (see recipe, page 236)

1 small handful flat-leaf parsley, roughly chopped

Extra-virgin olive oil, to serve

DRESSING

3 Tbsp apple cider vinegar

1 Tbsp honey (optional)

1 tsp Dijon mustard

Sea salt and freshly ground black pepper

Heat the coconut oil in a frying pan over medium heat. Add the bacon and cook until golden and crisp, 5 to 8 minutes. Strain the bacon fat from the pan into a bowl and reserve. Set the cooked bacon aside, keeping warm.

To make the dressing, combine the vinegar, honey (if using), and mustard with the reserved bacon fat and mix well. Season with a little salt and pepper. Keep warm.

Place the iceberg wedges on a platter and spoon on the dressing. Scatter over the bacon and egg, then drizzle on the mayonnaise, sprinkle over the parsley, and finish with a splash of olive oil.

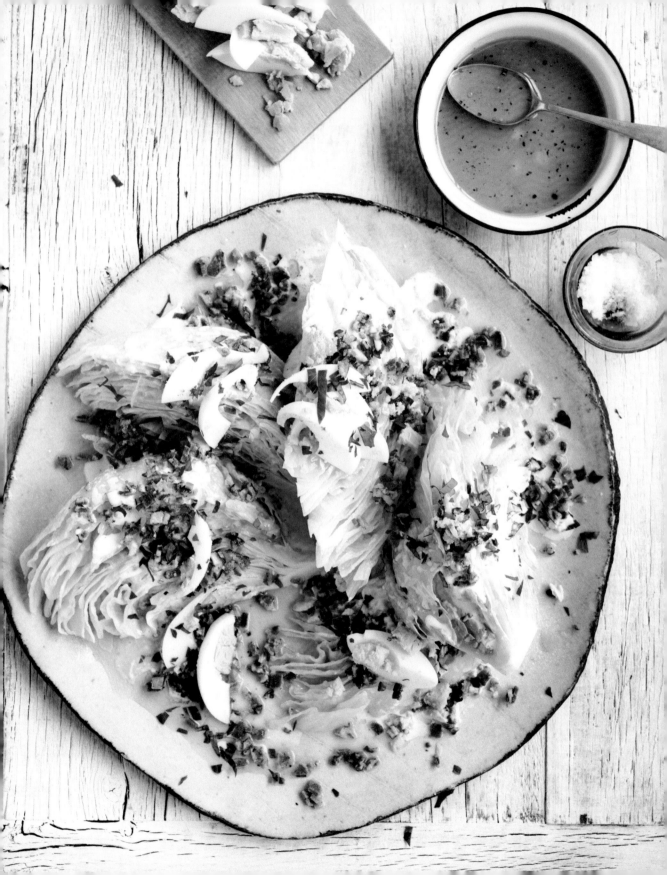

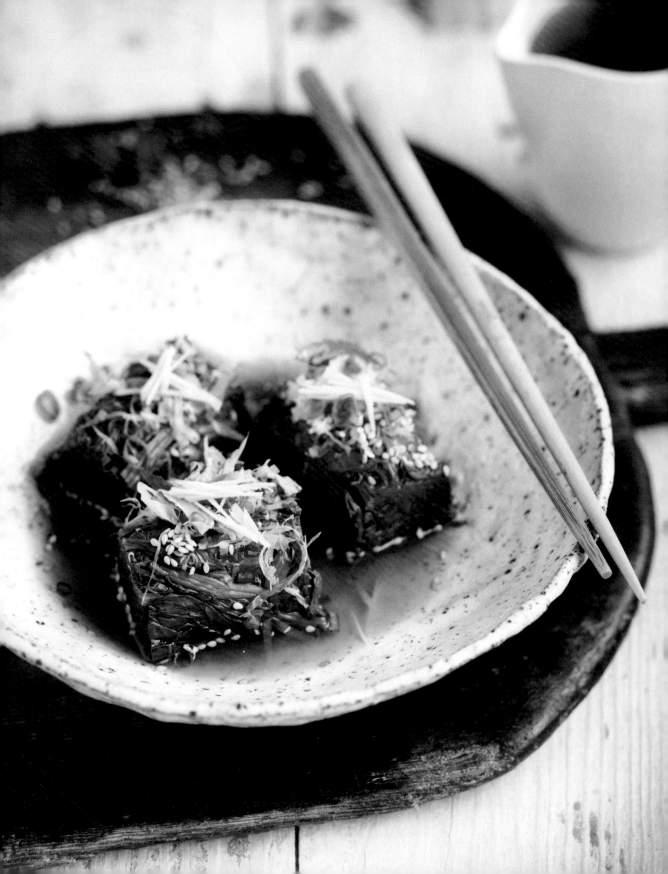

JAPANESE SPINACH SALAD (OHITASHI)

Pete ate this dish the first time he went to a Japanese restaurant close to 30 years ago—and he can still remember the taste, texture, and sheer amazement at how good spinach could be. He has kept this as true to tradition as he could and, to be honest, he doesn't think there is anything he can do to improve it. When you feel like being Popeye and upping your spinach intake, serve this alongside basically anything: soups, stir-fries, grilled seafood and meat, or raw meat or seafood dishes.

Place the dashi, tamari, and coconut sugar (if using) in a small saucepan and heat, stirring, until the broth is warm and the sugar dissolves. Remove from the heat and set aside until needed.

Blanch the spinach in a large saucepan of boiling salted water for 10 seconds until wilted and bright green. Drain and plunge into ice water to cool completely. Drain again and squeeze out as much water as possible.

Fill another small saucepan with water and bring to a boil. Add the ginger and cook for 3 minutes, until softened slightly. Drain and allow to cool.

Using a bamboo sushi mat and working at the edge closest to you, pack and mold the spinach into a long cylinder shape about 1 inch thick and roll up tightly. Carefully unroll and remove the mat. Alternatively, if you don't have a sushi mat, simply shape the spinach into a long, 1-inch-thick cylinder. Use a sharp knife to cut the spinach into 1½-inch lengths.

Divide the spinach between 2 serving bowls, ladle over the broth, then finish with the spring onion, ginger, and bonito flakes. Drizzle over a couple of drops of sesame oil and serve.

Serves: 2

1 cup cold dashi

1 Tbsp tamari or coconut aminos

1 tsp coconut sugar (optional)

4 bunches English spinach, stalks trimmed and discarded

¾-inch piece ginger, cut into thin matchsticks

TO SERVE:

1 whole spring onion, green part thinly sliced

2 Tbsp bonito flakes

Sesame oil

KALE CAESAR SALAD

This is Pete's favorite photo in this book. He won't say it is his favorite recipe because that is way too hard to pick! When he looks at this image, he just wants to eat this salad for breakfast, lunch, or dinner—because, seriously, that is when this dish can and should be eaten.

It makes the most gorgeous breakfast; it is basically bacon and eggs with some greens, which is one of Pete's favorite ways to start the day. It is also the perfect lunch to take to work or school, as it is filling and nutritious. And for dinner . . . well, it is perfect as it isn't too heavy and it's something that can be whipped up in under 15 minutes.

Serves: 4

6 to 8 rashers bacon

4 eggs

1 bunch kale, thinly sliced

Juice of 1 lemon

1 Tbsp extra-virgin olive oil

2 Tbsp chopped flat-leaf parsley leaves

2 Tbsp pine nuts, soaked and toasted

4 anchovy fillets, rinsed and halved (optional)

4 macadamia nuts, grated

CAESAR DRESSING

2 egg yolks

4 anchovy fillets, rinsed and finely chopped

1 garlic clove, crushed

1 Tbsp lemon juice

1 tsp Dijon mustard

1 cup light olive oil

Sea salt and freshly ground black pepper

Pan-fry the bacon until crisp and golden. Remove from the pan, drain on paper towel, and leave to cool. Chop into small pieces and set aside.

Place the eggs in a large saucepan of water. Bring to a boil over medium heat and simmer for 5 minutes or until cooked to your liking. Remove from the heat, drain, and cool in ice water. Peel, quarter, and set aside.

Place the kale in a bowl and add the lemon juice and olive oil. Mix gently, rubbing the lemon juice and oil into the kale, and allow to stand for 5 minutes.

TO MAKE THE CAESAR DRESSING, combine the egg yolks, anchovies, garlic, lemon juice, and mustard in a food processor or blender. Process briefly until combined. With the motor running, begin to gradually add the oil, drop by drop, until the dressing has emulsified and thickened slightly. Now pour in the remaining oil in a steady stream and continue to process until the dressing is the consistency of heavy cream. Check the seasoning, adding salt and pepper or more lemon juice as desired.

Place half the dressing on the kale and mix gently.

Tip the dressed kale into a large serving bowl and scatter on the parsley, pine nuts, and anchovies (if using). Top the salad with the bacon, quartered eggs, and grated macadamia nuts.

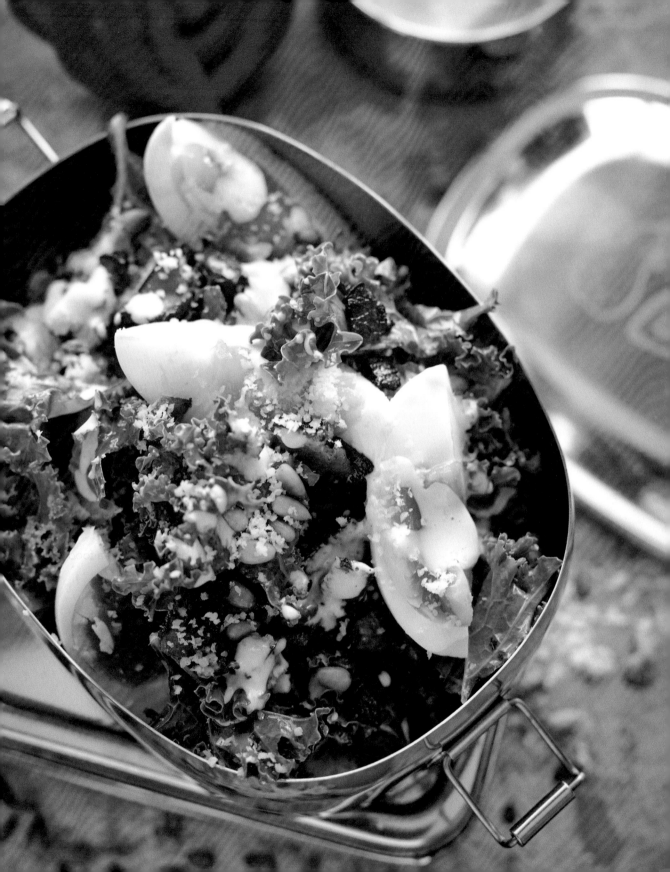

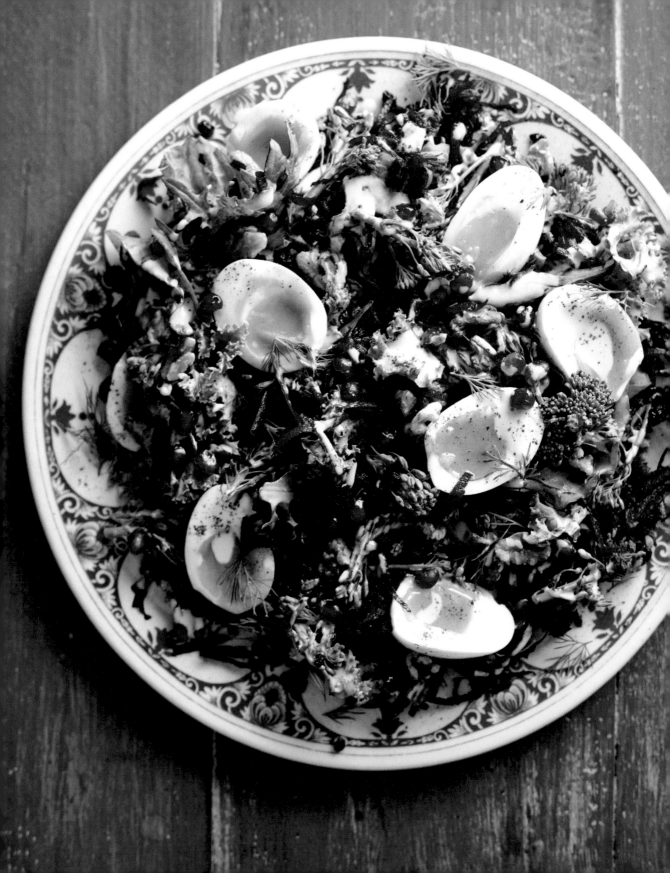

RAW BEET SALAD

When does a salad become a meal in itself? When it is nutritionally balanced with good sources of fat and protein and it leaves you feeling satiated. And that is exactly what this salad does.

Place all the ingredients in a large bowl. Add dressing (if using) and gently toss until everything is evenly coated. Season with salt and pepper.

Arrange the salad on a platter, then top with the eggs. Season with more salt or pepper, if desired.

Serves: 3 or 4 as a main course

1 large beet, grated

½ bunch frisée, leaves separated

1 bunch broccolini, woody ends trimmed, thinly sliced

4 stalks kale, stalks discarded and leaves torn

3 Tbsp roughly chopped walnuts, activated (i.e., soaked 4 to 8 hours in salted water)

1 large handful mixed fresh herbs (such as mint, flat-leaf parsley, dill, and chervil)

Seeds of ¼ pomegranate

3 Tbsp goji berries (optional)

Dressing (optional)

TO SERVE:

4 hard-boiled eggs, peeled and halved

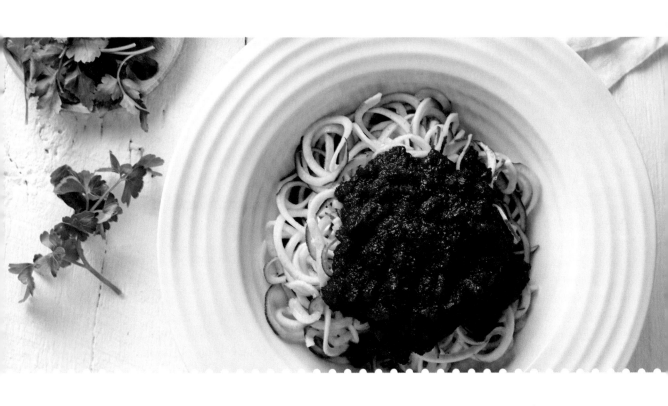

MEALS

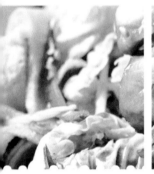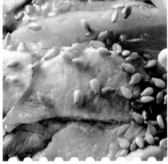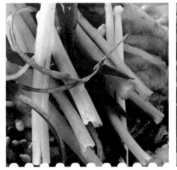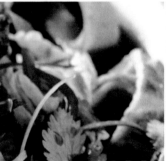

BRAISED GINGER CHICKEN

Ginger has been used for centuries to aid digestion; to help with nausea, morning sickness, and travel sickness; and to reduce muscle stiffness and pain. Here is a wonderful, warming dish for the whole family. You cut a whole chicken into pieces, but feel free to substitute just thighs (with the skin on), breasts, drumsticks, or the thigh and leg together.

Serves: 4 to 6

4 lb chicken, cut into 8 pieces

1 Tbsp tapioca flour (optional)

3 Tbsp coconut oil or good-quality animal fat, melted

1 onion, chopped

4 garlic cloves, finely sliced

2-inch piece ginger, cut into thin strips

Sea salt and freshly ground black pepper

½ cup dry white wine

1 cup Chicken Bone Broth (see recipe, page 87)

1 Tbsp fish sauce

1 Tbsp tamari or coconut aminos

3 long red chilies, seeded and finely sliced (leave some seeds in if you like extra heat)

4 spring onions, cut into thin strips

1 bunch bok choy, trimmed

Preheat the oven to 325°F.

Place the chicken pieces in a large bowl, add the tapioca flour (if using), and toss to coat.

Melt the oil in a roasting pan over medium-high heat. Add the onion and cook, stirring occasionally, for 5 minutes, until translucent. Stir in the garlic and ginger and cook for 1 minute until fragrant. Add the chicken pieces, skin side down, season with salt and pepper, and cook for 3 minutes until lightly golden.

Pour in the wine, broth, fish sauce, and tamari and scatter on the chilies and spring onion.

Cover the pan tightly with a double layer of foil and braise in the oven for 45 minutes. Remove from the oven and mix in the bok choy. Cover and return to the oven for 15 minutes, until the chicken is cooked through.

Season the sauce if needed and serve the braised chicken with a side of Asian greens such as bok choy, choy sum, Chinese broccoli, or water spinach.

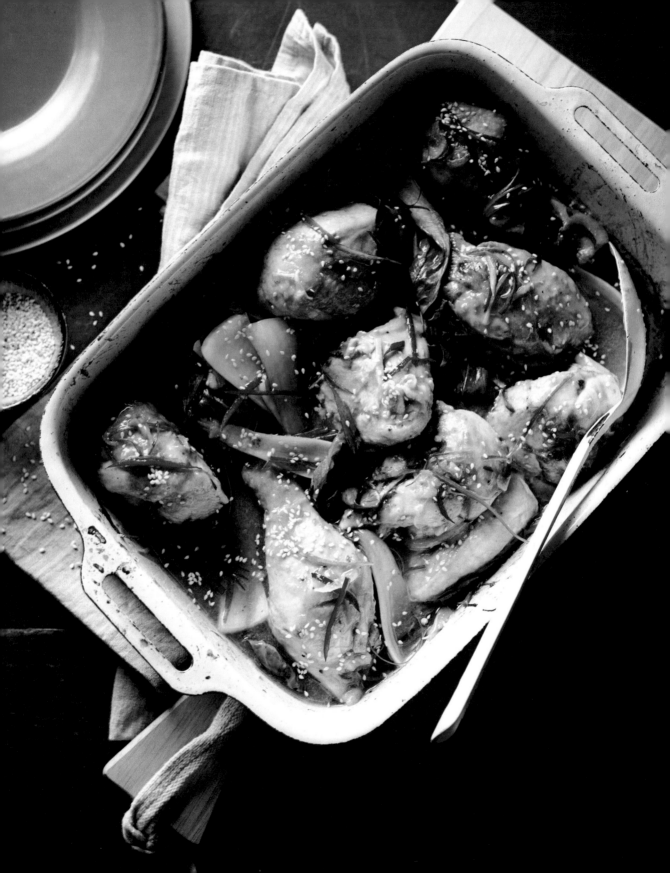

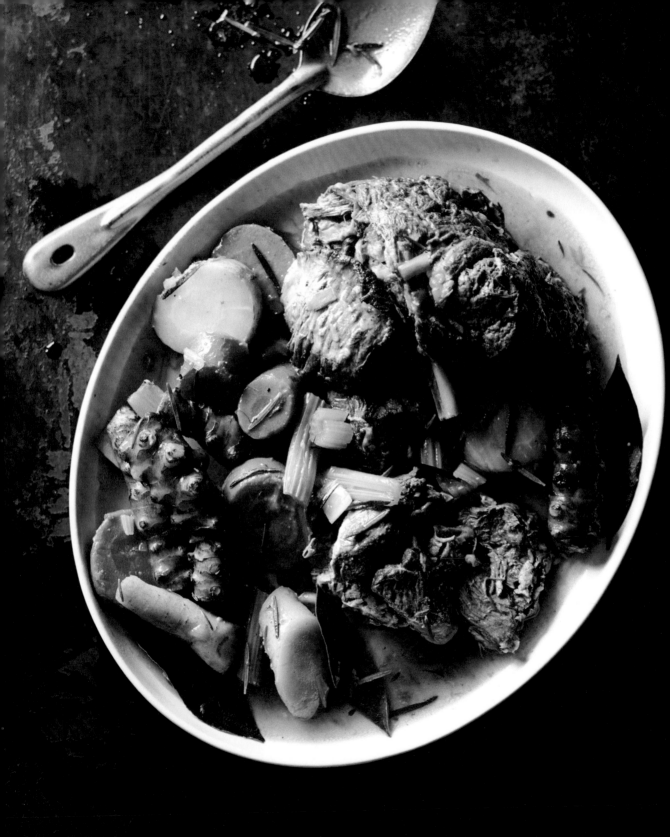

BRAISED LAMB WITH JERUSALEM ARTICHOKES

Is there a more magnificent pairing than cumin and lamb? Whether it is a simple lamb burger patty with ground cumin or a braised lamb shoulder with cumin seeds, the flavor combination creates lasting memories. Here, lamb and cumin are teamed with Jerusalem artichokes, one of Pete's all-time favorite ingredients. If you can't find Jerusalem artichokes, use sweet potatoes, turnips, parsnips, or fennel.

Preheat the oven to 200°F or the lowest setting.

Score the fat of the lamb and rub the cumin seeds, salt, and pepper into the score marks.

Melt the oil in a large flameproof casserole dish over medium-high heat, add the lamb in batches, and brown on all sides for a total of 3 to 5 minutes. Remove from the dish and place, fat side up, on a plate.

Add the onion to the casserole dish and cook, stirring occasionally, for 2 to 4 minutes, until softened. Add the carrots, celery, and garlic and cook until the vegetables start to color, 2 to 4 minutes.

Stir in the wine, broth, rosemary, bay leaves, and celery seeds, bring to a boil, and season with salt and pepper. Then return the browned lamb to the dish along with the parsnips and Jerusalem artichokes.

Cover the dish with a lid or tightly seal with foil and braise in the oven for 10 to 11 hours, until the lamb pulls apart easily. Serve with a crisp green salad.

Serves: 4 to 6

5 lb lamb leg (bone in), cut into 5-inch pieces (ask your butcher to do this)

1 tsp cumin seeds

Sea salt and freshly ground black pepper

1 Tbsp coconut oil or good-quality animal fat

1 large onion, roughly chopped

3 carrots, roughly chopped

2 celery stalks, roughly chopped

6 garlic cloves, roughly chopped

1 cup dry white wine

¾ cup Chicken Bone Broth (see recipe, page 87)

3 sprigs rosemary, leaves only

2 bay leaves

1 tsp celery seeds

4 parsnips, cut into thirds

4 Jerusalem artichokes, halved

CAULIFLOWER AND BACON TOAST WITH AVOCADO AND FRIED EGG

This cauliflower and bacon toast is super simple to prepare and will make your bread craving a thing of the past. Pete has teamed the cauliflower toast with egg and avocado, which makes for a perfect meal anytime.

Serves: 4

1½ Tbsp coconut oil or good-quality animal fat

4 eggs

1 avocado, sliced

1 handful watercress

1 tsp chili oil (optional)

1 lemon, cut into wedges

CAULIFLOWER AND BACON TOAST

¼ head cauliflower, chopped into small pieces

1½ Tbsp coconut oil

Sea salt and freshly ground black pepper

2 rashers rindless bacon, finely diced

2 eggs

Preheat the oven to 400°F. Line a baking tray with parchment paper.

TO MAKE THE CAULIFLOWER AND BACON TOAST, place the cauliflower in the bowl of a food processor and process to fine crumbs. Melt 1 tablespoon of the coconut oil in a large frying pan over medium heat. Add the cauliflower crumbs and cook for 4 to 6 minutes, until softened. Season with salt and pepper, transfer to a large bowl, and allow to cool. Wipe the pan clean, add the remaining oil, and fry the bacon over medium-high heat until light golden, about 3 to 4 minutes. Allow to cool. Transfer the cooled bacon to the cauliflower, add the eggs, and mix to combine. Season with salt and pepper. Spoon 2 tablespoons of the cauliflower mixture onto the prepared tray and gently spread out to form a patty, approximately 3 inches in diameter. Repeat, allowing ¾ inch between each patty, until all of the mixture is used and you have 4 patties in total. Bake for 15 to 20 minutes until golden and crisp.

To complete the recipe, heat the oil or fat in a frying pan over medium heat. Crack the eggs into the pan (if the pan is not big enough to cook all the eggs at once, cook them in batches). Cook the eggs for 2½ to 3 minutes, or to your liking. Season with salt and pepper.

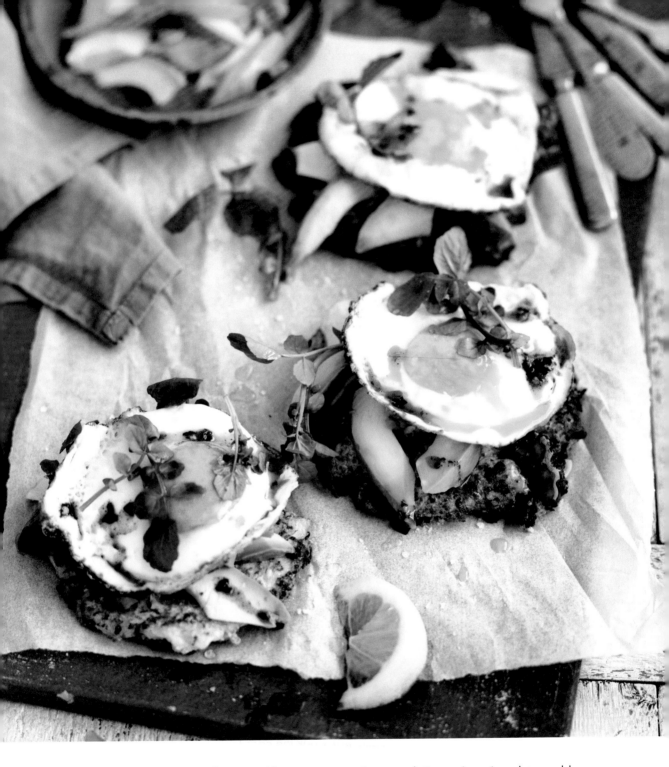

To serve, transfer the cauliflower and bacon toast patties to a platter or 4 serving plates, add a few slices of avocado to each, then slide an egg on top. Sprinkle on a few sprigs of watercress, add some chili oil, if desired, and place lemon wedges on the side.

CHICKEN LIVER PÂTÉ

We need to eat more offal. And pâté is the easiest and most subtle way to add it—in the form of liver—to your diet. In Pete's house, they absolutely love liver and eat it at least three times a week. They make a big batch of pâté or terrine, then freeze it in small jars or portions so they can enjoy it as part of a meal, as a snack, or as an amazing lunchtime treat.

They like to serve theirs with raw vegetables—like carrots, cucumber, celery, fennel, and salad greens—and paleo bread or seed and nut crackers with gherkins and fermented vegetables on the side. You can also use it in lettuce wraps or try adding a spoonful to your chicken soup or Bolognese sauce just before serving.

Serves: 4 to 6

2 Tbsp duck fat, tallow, or coconut oil, melted

1 onion, chopped

4 garlic cloves, chopped

1½ tsp thyme leaves

2 bay leaves

4 sage leaves, chopped

½ cup red wine (such as shiraz)

1 lb chicken livers, trimmed

1 Tbsp Dijon mustard

½ cup bone marrow, duck fat, tallow, or lard, melted

¼ cup Chicken Bone Broth (see recipe, page 87)

Sea salt and freshly ground black pepper

Place 1 tablespoon of the fat, the onion, garlic, and thyme in a saucepan over medium-low heat and cook, stirring occasionally, for 10 to 15 minutes, until the onion is softened and slightly caramelized. Add the bay leaves and sage, pour in the wine, and simmer until mixture is reduced to a glaze. Set aside to cool. Remove the bay leaves.

Heat the remaining fat in a large frying pan over medium-high heat, add the livers in batches, and cook for about 30 seconds on each side, until they are brown but still pink in the middle. Remove from the pan and set aside to cool.

Place the cooked livers, onion-wine reduction, mustard, marrow, and broth in a blender and blend until smooth. Add salt to taste and blend a few times to mix through.

Pass the pâté through a fine sieve and add pepper to taste.

Spoon the pâté into jars or bowls, leaving ½ inch of space at the top. Cover and place in the refrigerator for 4 to 6 hours to set.

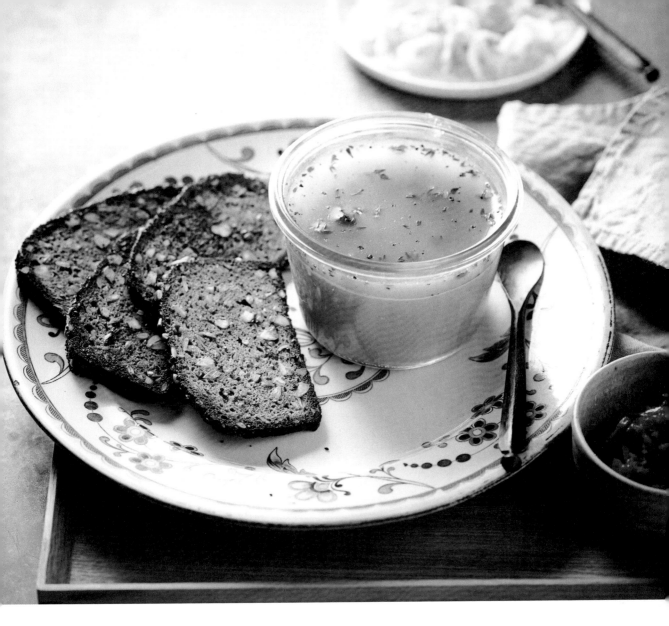

FOR THE JELLY, combine the thyme and broth in a saucepan, bring to a boil, and simmer until reduced by half. Meanwhile, sprinkle the gelatin over 3 tablespoons of water and set aside for 2 minutes. Add to the hot broth and stir until dissolved. Allow to cool completely before pouring over the pâtés. Chill for 1 hour before serving.

Serve the pâté with toasted seed and nut loaf, paleo bread, or seeded crackers of your choice and sauerkraut.

JELLY

4 thyme sprigs, leaves only

1 cup Chicken Bone Broth (see page 87)

½ Tbsp powdered gelatin

TO SERVE:

Seed and nut loaf or paleo bread, toasted, or seeded crackers

Sauerkraut (see recipe, page 126)

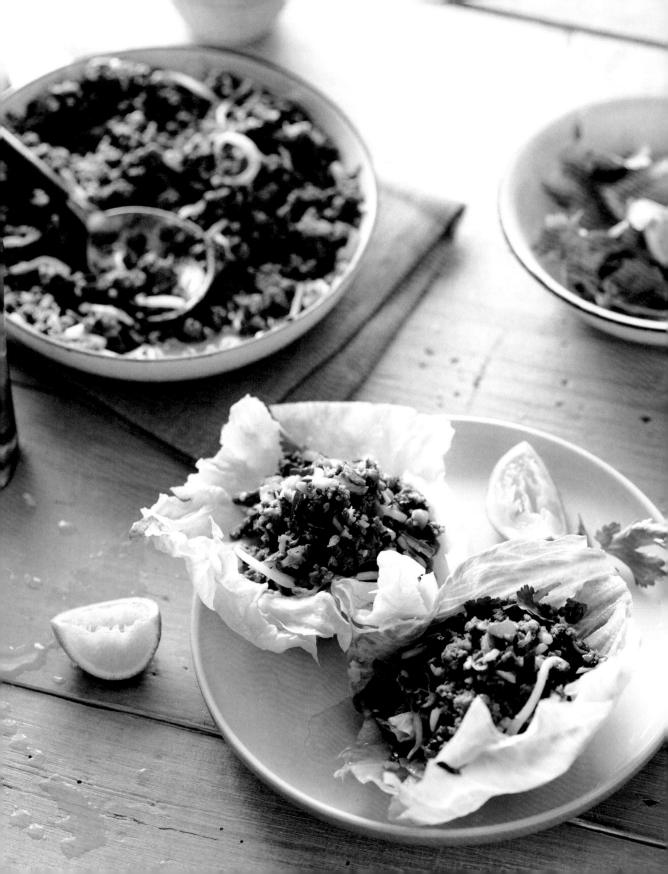

CHICKEN SAN CHOY BAU

Has there ever been a more family-oriented dish than the classic lettuce wraps? Let's get to the heart of this recipe: you have as much creative freedom as possible. It's recommended to start with base aromatics (such as garlic, ginger, coriander root, spring onion, and tamari) as the foundation, and then play around with different proteins (such as grass-fed beef, chicken, lamb, duck, quail, pork, lobster, crab, or a combination of any of these) that are mixed with water chestnuts and mushrooms.

Feel free to add bean sprouts, loads of herbs, water spinach, kale, cauliflower, asparagus . . . This is how you create recipes, with an open mind and palate.

Heat a wok or large frying pan over medium-high heat. When hot, add the oil and swirl around the wok. Add the garlic, shallots, and ginger and cook for 1 minute. Add the chicken and mushrooms and cook for another 4 to 5 minutes, stirring occasionally, until cooked through and browned. Add the tamari, fish sauce, and honey, if using, and toss to mix. Add the water chestnuts, spring onions, and chilies and keep stirring until the mixture is well combined.

Cook until heated through (2 to 3 minutes). Remove from the heat, mix in the bean sprouts, and check seasoning, adding more fish sauce or some sea salt if needed.

To serve, place the lettuce leaves on four plates. Top each lettuce leaf with some of the chicken mixture and garnish with coriander leaves and lime wedges. (Alternatively, place the lettuce leaves on a large, communal serving platter and let everyone assemble the dish themselves.)

Serves: 4

1 Tbsp coconut oil, tallow, duck fat, or other good-quality fat

3 cloves garlic, minced

4 shallots, chopped

2 tsp peeled and grated fresh ginger

2½ cups ground free-range chicken

1½ cups shiitake mushrooms, chopped

2 Tbsp wheat-free tamari

1 Tbsp fish sauce, plus more to serve

1 Tbsp raw honey (optional)

1 cup water chestnuts, drained and finely chopped

4 spring onions, finely chopped

1 or 2 fresh long red chilies, seeded and chopped

1 cup bean sprouts

8 iceberg lettuce leaves, washed and dried

Fresh coriander leaves, torn, to serve

Lime wedges, to serve

CRACKLING CHICKEN

Pete loves the simplicity of this cooking technique, and he also loves to cook duck breast this way so it gets really crispy skin. Serve with a generous salad or cooked green vegetables and some fermented veggies for good measure.

Serves: 4

8 chicken thigh fillets, skin left on

1 Tbsp sea salt

2 tsp coconut oil or other good-quality fat

2 tsp spice mix of your choice (Pete likes a Cajun or Moroccan mix)

Lemon wedges, to serve

Flatten the chicken thighs with a mallet to ensure they cook evenly. Season the skin with salt.

Melt the oil in a large, heavy frying pan over medium-high heat. Place four of the chicken thighs, skin side down, in the hot pan and season the exposed side with 1 teaspoon of the spice mix. If your seasoning doesn't include salt, you may wish to add a little.

Fry the chicken, undisturbed, for 6 to 8 minutes, until crispy and golden brown. Flip the chicken over and fry for 3 minutes, until cooked through. Remove from the pan and keep warm. Repeat with the remaining chicken.

Serve with lemon wedges and vegetables or salad.

TIP: If you are using duck, cook it over very low heat for 12 to 16 minutes to allow the fat to render and give you the most amazingly crispy skin.

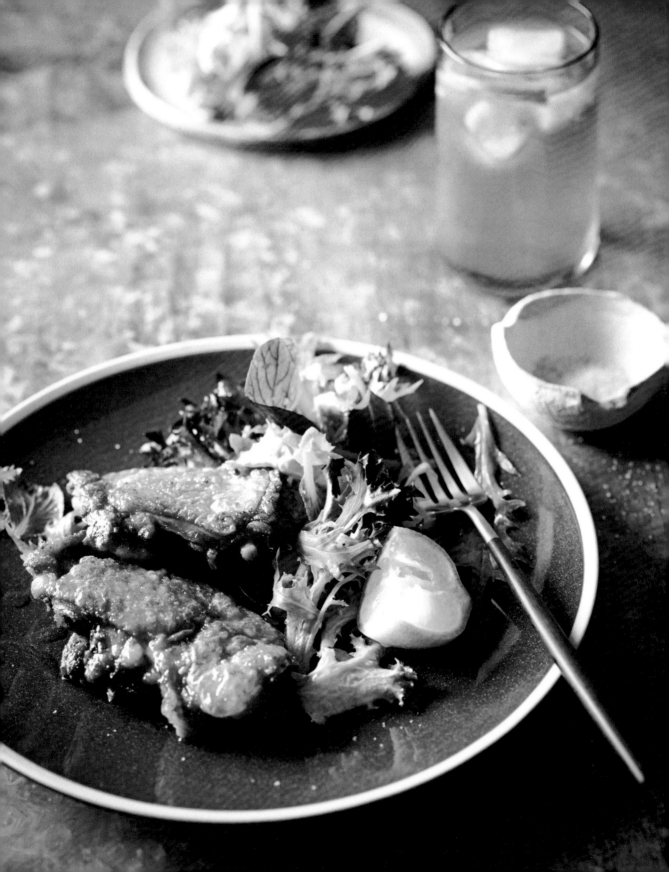

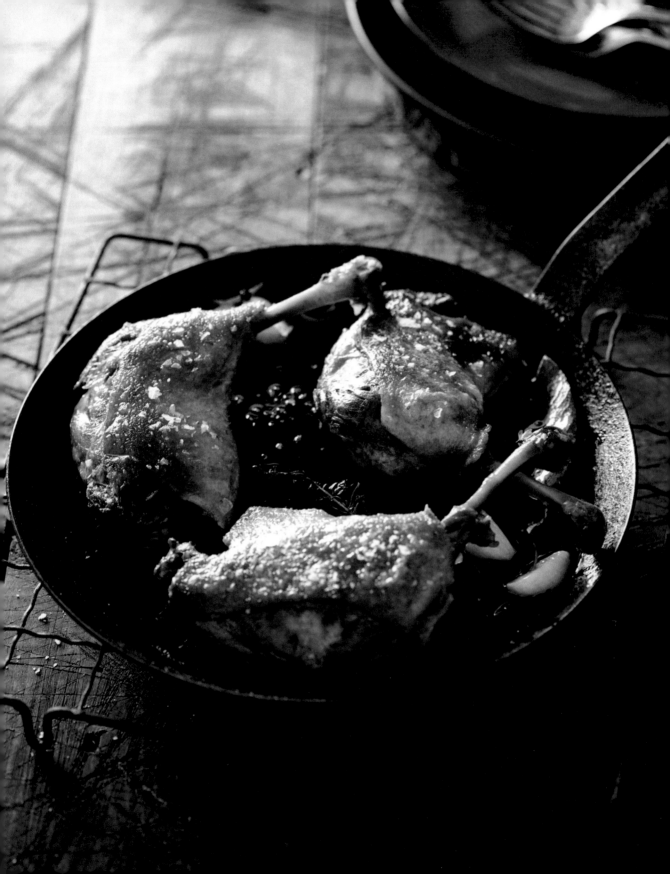

CRISPY DUCK CONFIT

Recently, Pete cooked up some leftover duck confit for breakfast with some greens and cabbage. It was the best culinary start to his day ever! He decided then and there that he would never again eat a boring dish for breakfast. Now his breakfasts feature curries, roasts, braises, soups, or leftovers from the night before. You'll need to begin this recipe 2 days ahead.

Combine the salt, juniper berries, orange zest, and orange juice in a large, shallow bowl and mix well. Rub the salt mixture into the duck to evenly coat. Cover with plastic wrap and refrigerate for 12 hours or, for best results, 24 hours.

Preheat the oven to 225°F.

Rinse the duck legs, then pat dry with a paper towel. Place the duck legs in a single layer in a casserole dish. Add the thyme, bay leaves, and garlic and pour on the fat to completely cover the duck legs.

Bake the duck legs in the oven for 2 hours, until very tender. Allow the duck confit to cool completely at room temperature, then refrigerate overnight.

When ready to crisp the duck legs, preheat the oven to 425°F. Remove the duck legs from the fat and pat dry with a paper towel, being careful not to break the skin. Reserve the fat for another use.

Arrange the duck legs in a single layer in a lightly greased roasting pan and bake in the oven for 20 to 25 minutes, until golden. Sprinkle with a little salt, if needed, and serve with your favorite salad or side.

Serves: 4

4 Tbsp fine sea salt

1 Tbsp juniper berries

1 tsp finely grated orange zest

2 Tbsp orange juice

4 duck legs

5 thyme sprigs

4 bay leaves

4 whole garlic cloves

3½ cups duck or goose fat or other good-quality animal fat, melted

GRASS-FED STEAK
WITH CHIMICHURRI
AND BONE MARROW

All around the world in so many cuisines, we see similar philosophies that promote the use of simple and honest ingredients. Nothing sums this up more than the classic and versatile chimichurri, an Argentinean condiment that is a beautiful balance of fresh and dried herbs, chili, spices, vinegar or lemon juice, and oil. Thailand has its own version, the classic nam jim, Vietnam has nuoc cham, Italy has salsa verde, France has its gribiche, and Spain has its escabeche, to name just a few. Pete sees chimichurri as one of the easiest ways to elevate a gorgeous piece of grass-fed steak or wild-caught fish or grilled mushrooms.

Serves: 8

4 grass-fed sirloin, filet mignon, or ribeye steaks (about 7 oz each)

3 Tbsp coconut oil

Sea salt and freshly ground black pepper

3½ oz beef marrow (no bone), chopped

Chimichurri (see recipe opposite)

Lemon wedges, to serve

Remove the steaks from the refrigerator at least 15 minutes before cooking so they come to room temperature. Heat the pan or a grill plate to hot.

Coat the steaks with a little coconut oil and season with salt and pepper. Cook the steaks for 2½ to 3 minutes, or until browned, then flip them over and cook for another 2½ to 3 minutes (for medium-rare). Remove from the heat and place on a plate, cover with foil, and let them rest in a warm place for 4 minutes.

Return the pan to medium heat. Add the chopped marrow and cook for 1 minute, until lightly golden and cooked through. Season with salt and pepper, then add to the chimichurri and stir to combine.

Spoon some chimichurri with bone marrow over each steak and serve with a seasonal salad of your choice and a wedge of lemon.

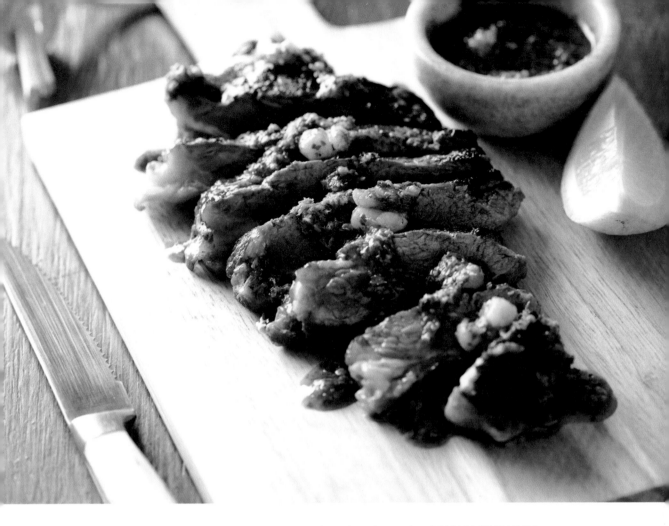

Place the garlic and a little salt in a mortar and crush with a pestle. Add the jalapeño, parsley, and coriander and pound to a paste. Stir in the vinegar, cumin, and oil, then taste and season with salt and pepper. (You could also make the chimichurri in a food processor.)

CHIMICHURRI

Makes: ¾ cup

3 garlic cloves, peeled

Sea salt

1 jalapeño or long red chili, seeded and finely chopped

1 very large handful flat-leaf parsley leaves

1 very large handful coriander leaves

3 Tbsp apple cider vinegar

½ tsp ground cumin

3 Tbsp olive oil or coconut oil

Freshly ground black pepper

GRASS-FED BEEF CARPACCIO WITH CELERIAC RÉMOULADE

Carpaccio is a delicious dish of thinly sliced raw beef—usually fillet or sirloin—seasoned with olive oil, lemon juice, salt, pepper, and that is about it. Celeriac rémoulade, a combination of thinly sliced celeriac and mustard mayonnaise, is to die for and works well on its own. However, when you pair it with carpaccio, all nutritional bases are covered, and you get this amazing textural experience from the aioli, the crunchy celeriac, and the melt-in-your-mouth beef.

Serves: 4

4 grass-fed beef tenderloins (about 2½ oz each)

2 Tbsp extra-virgin olive oil, plus extra to serve

1 lemon, halved

Sea salt and freshly ground black pepper

1 large handful wild arugula leaves

1 tsp snipped chives, to serve

1 small handful chervil sprigs, to serve

Finely grated fresh horseradish, to serve

CELERIAC RÉMOULADE

½ celeriac, julienned

2 tsp whole-grain mustard

2 Tbsp chopped flat-leaf parsley leaves

4 Tbsp Aioli (see recipe, page 254)

1 tsp truffle-infused olive oil (optional)

Sea salt and freshly ground black pepper

TO MAKE THE CELERIAC RÉMOULADE, combine all the ingredients in a bowl.

Place one piece of beef between two sheets of plastic wrap and pound with a meat mallet until $1/16$ inch thick. Remove the top layer of plastic wrap, flip the beef over onto a serving plate, and remove the remaining layer of plastic wrap. Drizzle on 2 teaspoons of the olive oil and a squeeze of lemon juice, and gently rub in with your fingertips. Repeat this process with the remaining beef, olive oil, and lemon juice. Season with salt and pepper.

For each serving, use 2 tablespoons to shape a large spoonful of celeriac rémoulade into an oval (quenelle) and place on the beef. Scatter one-quarter of the arugula, chives, and chervil on each plate, then drizzle with some extra olive oil. Finish with grated horseradish.

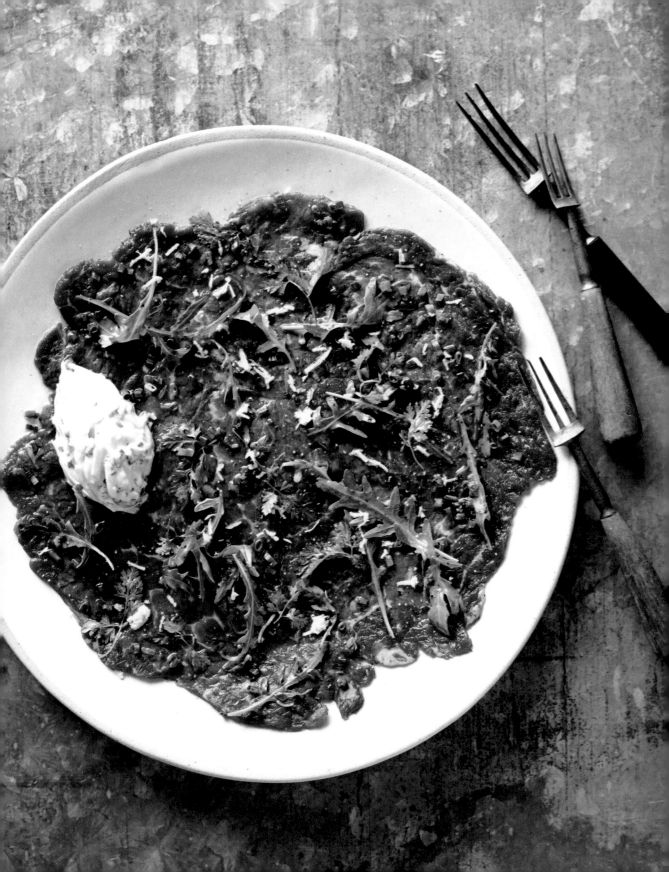

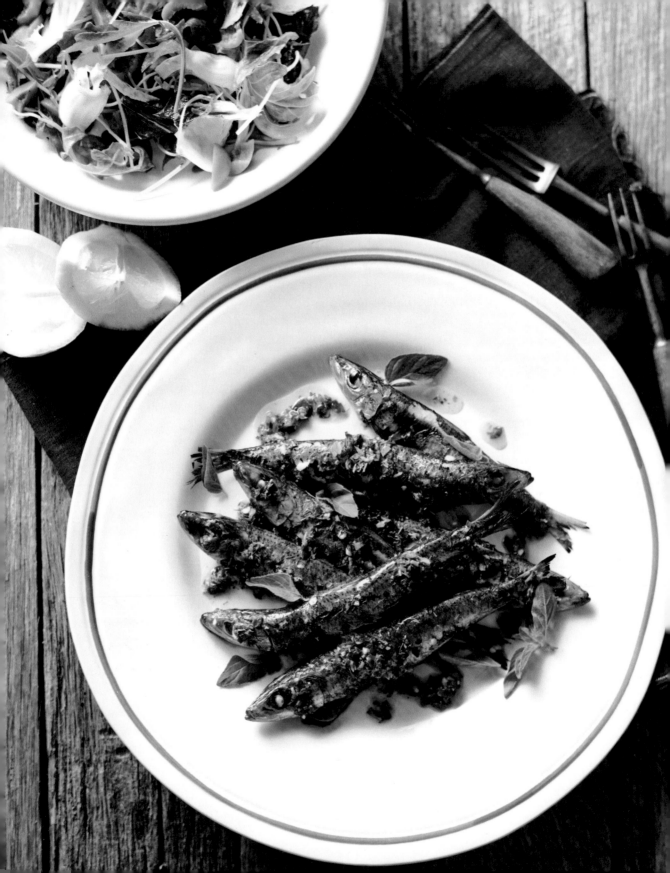

GRILLED SARDINES
WITH CHILI, OREGANO, AND LEMON

Sardines really should appear more on people's tables. Aside from the awesome health benefits of their calcium, omega-3s, and other goodies, sardines are a sustainable seafood. This recipe is a great way to introduce your family to sardines: grilled on the barbecue with a delicious marinade, and served with a gorgeous crisp salad and some fermented vegetables.

To make the marinade, mix all ingredients together.

Brush some of the marinade over the sardines (keep the rest for drizzling).

Heat a barbecue plate or grill pan to hot. Cook the sardines on each side for 40 to 60 seconds, until just cooked through. Drizzle over some of the remaining marinade, scatter on the oregano leaves, and serve with the lemon wedges and a salad.

Serves: 2 to 4

10 whole sardines, cleaned and rinsed (ask your fishmonger to do this)

Oregano leaves, to serve

Lemon wedges, to serve

MARINADE

Scant ½ cup coconut oil, melted

2 Tbsp dried oregano

2 Tbsp chopped fresh oregano leaves

1 tsp chili flakes

2 Tbsp chopped flat-leaf parsley leaves

Finely grated zest of 1 lemon

1 garlic clove, finely chopped

Sea salt and freshly ground black pepper

HAM, EGG, AND MAYO LETTUCE WRAPS

With this tasty sandwich Pete has used lettuce as the wraps, but feel free to use coconut tortillas for a true sandwich. Please source the best-quality pastured ham you can spend your hard-earned cash on. If you avoid pork, replace it with cooked tuna or salmon. Or simply chop up all the ingredients with some avocado to make a killer salad!

Serves: 2

2 hard-boiled eggs, chopped

2 Tbsp mayonnaise (to make your own, see recipe below)

Sea salt and freshly ground black pepper

2 large romaine lettuce leaves

4 thin slices ham

1 carrot, grated

1 cucumber, peeled, seeded, and sliced

1 beet, peeled and grated (wear gloves to avoid staining hands)

MAYONNAISE

1 egg

2 egg yolks

1 tsp Dijon mustard

½ tsp fine sea salt

1 Tbsp apple cider vinegar

1 Tbsp lemon juice

2 cups olive oil or macadamia oil

Mix the hard-boiled eggs and the mayonnaise until well combined; season with salt and pepper.

Place two sheets of parchment paper on a work surface or cutting board and put a lettuce leaf on each sheet. Equally divide the ham, carrot, cucumber, beet, and egg mixture among the lettuce leaves, then roll up, wrap tightly, and cut in half.

FOR THE MAYONNAISE, place the egg, egg yolks, mustard, salt, vinegar, and lemon juice in a food processor and process for 1 to 2 minutes, until nice and smooth. With the motor running, slowly pour in the oil and process until it has emulsified and become thick and creamy.

Season with a little more salt if needed. Leftover mayo can be stored in an airtight container in the fridge for up to 4 days.

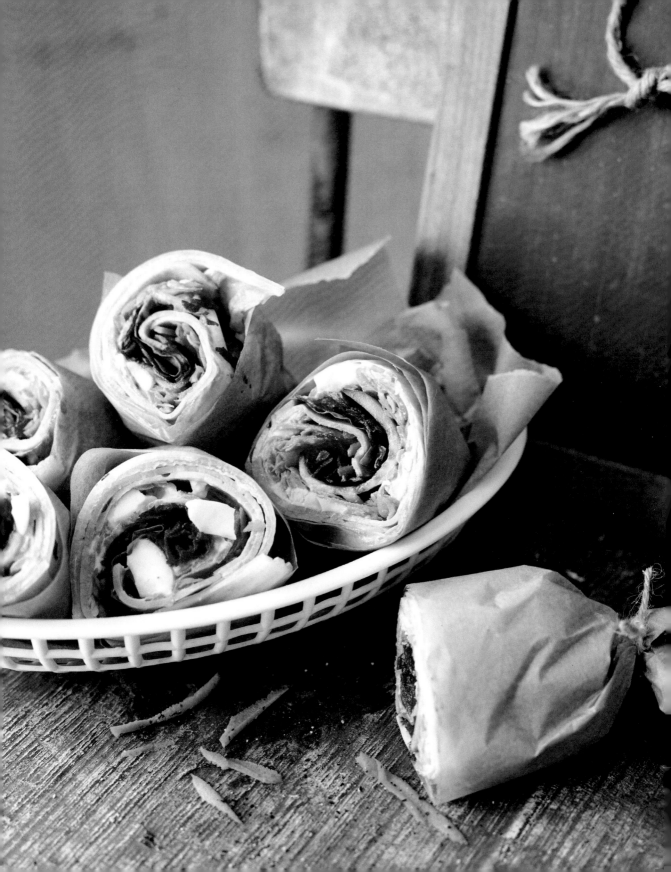

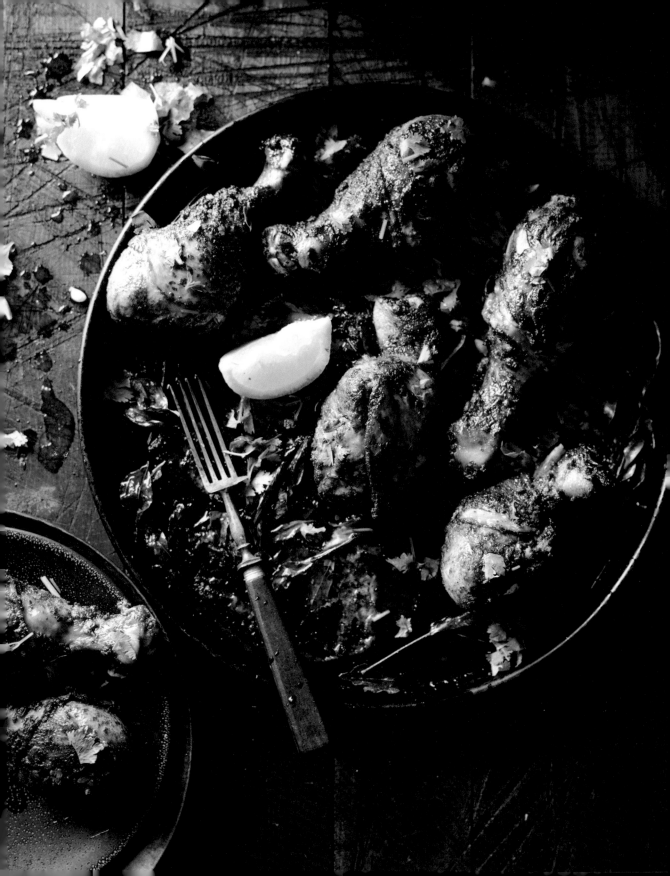

INDIAN-STYLE ROAST CHICKEN DRUMSTICKS

This recipe is special to Pete, as he made it with his friend Tony Coote. Tony, a biodynamic farmer who owns Mulloon Creek Natural Farms, isn't too confident in the kitchen—and Pete loved that because it meant he could show him how to create amazing-flavored dishes in a short time and with little fuss.

TO MAKE THE INDIAN SPICE DRY RUB, combine the coriander and cumin seeds in a dry frying pan and toast over medium heat until fragrant, 1 to 2 minutes. Remove from the heat and allow to cool. Grind the toasted seeds in a spice grinder or mortar and pestle. Mix the ground seeds with the remaining dry rub ingredients in a large bowl.

Add the chicken to the spice mix and massage until evenly coated. Cover the bowl with plastic wrap and refrigerate overnight or, for best results, for 24 hours so the flavors develop fully.

Preheat the oven to 350°F.

Brush the spiced drumsticks with the oil and arrange in a roasting pan in a single layer. Add 4 tablespoons of water. Roast for 40 minutes, turning halfway through cooking, until the chicken is cooked through and golden. Taste and season with salt and pepper, if needed.

Place the chicken on a large platter, then pour over the juices from the pan. Sprinkle with the coriander leaves and squeeze over the lemon juice.

Serves: 4

Indian Spice Dry Rub (see recipe below)

2½ lb chicken drumsticks

2 Tbsp coconut oil or other good-quality fat, melted

Sea salt and freshly ground black pepper

1 large handful coriander leaves, roughly chopped

Juice of 2 lemons

INDIAN SPICE DRY RUB

2 tsp coriander seeds

2 tsp cumin seeds

1 tsp sea salt

3 tsp ground turmeric

2½ tsp garam masala

½ tsp chili powder (or more if you like it spicy)

3 garlic cloves, finely chopped

2 Tbsp finely grated ginger

MOUTHWATERING MEATLOAF

Let's make meatloaf the most popular meal of the year. You can use this recipe as a starting point and then create your own version, taking inspiration from cuisines around the world. Experiment with herbs and spices and different proteins, and let your imagination run wild. Post your images on Instagram and Facebook with the headline "I'm bringing meatloaf back!" You might get a few weird comments from your friends, but Pete guarantees they will want the recipe once they've tried it.

Serves: 6 to 8

8 free-range bacon rashers, rind removed

2 Tbsp coconut oil or other good-quality fat

1 large onion, diced

1 small carrot, peeled and finely diced

2 celery stalks, finely chopped

2 garlic cloves, crushed

½ zucchini, seeded, peeled, and finely diced

1½ lb grass-fed ground beef

4 Tbsp coconut flour

4 Tbsp chopped flat-leaf parsley leaves

2 free-range organic eggs, lightly whisked

1 Tbsp Himalayan salt or sea salt

½ Tbsp freshly cracked black pepper

4 Tbsp Nomato Sauce (see recipe, page 239)

1 Tbsp honey (optional)

1 Tbsp apple cider vinegar

Preheat the oven to 350°F.

Line the base and sides of a 7" loaf pan with a piece of parchment paper, cutting into the corners to fit and allowing the paper to extend 2 inches above the rim. Line the base and sides of the prepared pan with five rashers of bacon, reserving the remaining rashers for the top.

Heat the oil in a frying pan over medium heat. Add the onion, carrot, and celery and cook for 5 minutes until softened, then add the garlic and zucchini and cook for another 3 minutes. Drain any excess liquid and allow the vegetables to cool completely in a colander.

Place the ground beef, coconut flour, parsley, cooked vegetables, eggs, salt, and pepper in a bowl and mix until well combined.

Pack the meat mixture firmly into the lined pan and lay the remaining bacon rashers on top, tucking them in so they don't overhang the sides of the pan. Bake for 25 minutes.

Meanwhile, to make a glaze, mix the Nomato Sauce, honey (if using), and vinegar in a small bowl. Remove the meatloaf from the oven and baste the top with the glaze. Return to the oven and continue cooking for another 25 minutes, until cooked through. To test for doneness, insert a thermometer into the center of the meatloaf—it should reach at least 160°F.

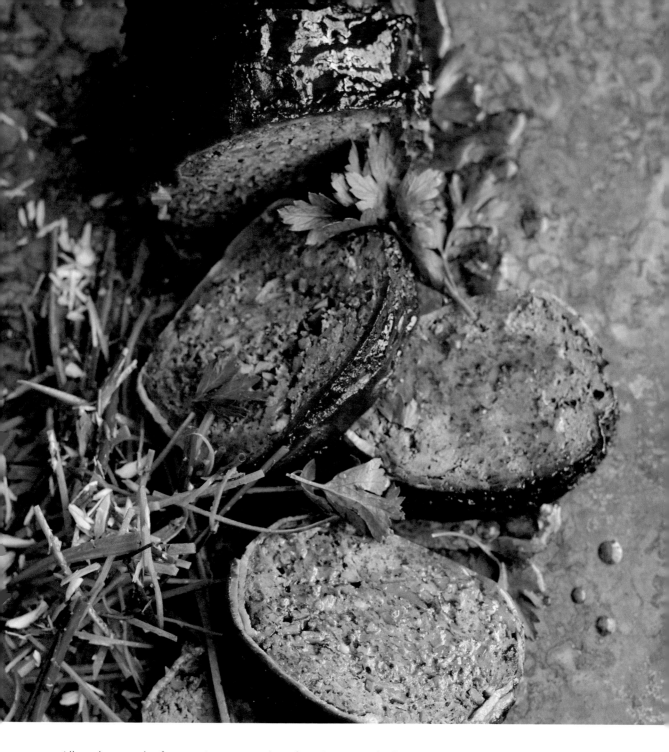

Allow the meatloaf to rest in a warm place for 10 minutes before turning it out of the pan; this will allow the meat to reabsorb any cooking liquids. Slice and serve with your favorite salad or roasted vegetables.

NOMATO SPAGHETTI BOLOGNESE

For everyone out there who loves a good beef ragu but can't tolerate tomatoes, Pete has created this wonderful Bolognese. The Nomato Sauce uses beets instead of tomato, which gives this dish a wonderful purple color along with some earthiness and sweetness. Serve with any type of spiral-cut vegetable, or try it with kelp noodles.

Serves 4

2 Tbsp coconut oil or good-quality animal fat

½ onion, finely chopped

3 garlic cloves, finely chopped

1⅓ lb ground beef

2 cups Nomato Sauce (see recipe, page 239)

1 tsp dried oregano

5 cups Chicken Bone Broth (see recipe, page 87)

Sea salt

5 zucchini or rutabaga, seeded, peeled, and spiral-cut into thin noodles

Splash olive oil

1 small handful basil or flat-leaf parsley leaves, chopped

Melt the coconut oil or other fat in a large frying pan over medium heat. Add the onion and garlic and cook, stirring, for 5 minutes, until soft. Add the beef and cook, stirring with a wooden spoon to break up any lumps, for another 5 minutes, until browned. Stir in the Nomato Sauce, oregano, 1 cup of the broth, and a good pinch of salt. Reduce the heat to low and simmer, stirring occasionally, for 20 minutes. Add a little more broth if the sauce is too thick.

Bring the remaining broth to a boil in a saucepan. Add the zucchini spaghetti and cook for 30 seconds, until tender. Drain, reserving the broth for another use. Toss the zucchini with the olive oil and season with salt.

Divide the zucchini among 4 serving bowls, spoon on the Bolognese sauce, sprinkle with the basil or parsley, and serve with vegetables or a salad.

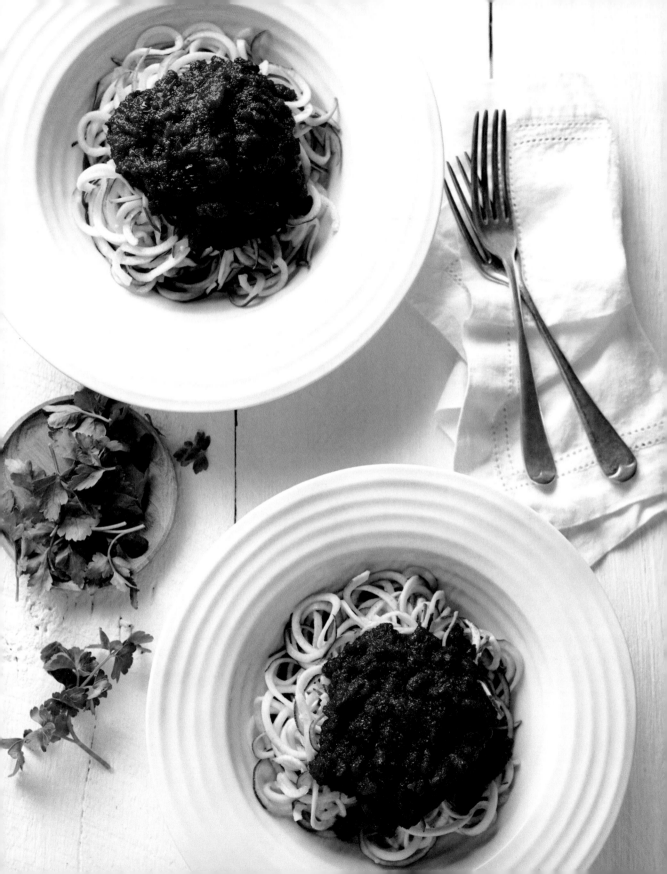

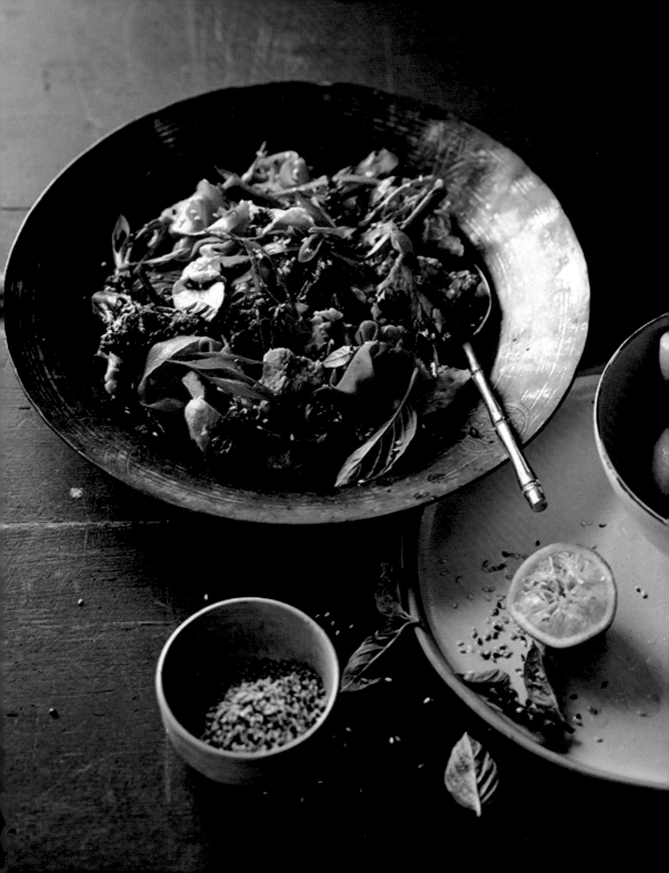

PAD SEE EW

Renowned author and paleo advocate Danielle Walker of the *Against All Grain* blog taught Pete this simple and delicious midweek family dinner. He visited Danielle to interview her and cook with her for his TV series. She was a a delight to work with; Pete loved her approach to cooking and we are sure you will, too. Thanks, Danielle, for the recipe, and keep inspiring millions of people.

To make carrot noodles, use the wide ribbon blade on a vegetable spiral-cut tool. Alternatively, place the carrots on a chopping board and, using a vegetable peeler, peel into thin, wide ribbons. (Save any leftover trimmings for broths or soups.)

Melt the oil in a wok or deep frying pan over medium heat. Add the garlic and chicken and stir-fry for 2 minutes, until the chicken changes color.

Add the broccolini and tamari to the pan and cook for another 5 minutes, until the broccolini is softened. Add the carrot noodles and stir-fry for another 3 minutes.

Push the stir-fry aside in the pan. Crack in the eggs, stir vigorously to scramble them, and cook for 2 minutes, until set. Mix everything in the pan together and serve immediately with the basil leaves and spring onion scattered over the top and the lime wedges on the side.

Serves: 4

5 peeled carrots

2 Tbsp coconut oil

6 garlic cloves, finely chopped

1⅓ lb chicken breast or thigh fillets, thinly sliced on the diagonal

1 lb broccolini, chopped into 2-inch lengths

4 Tbsp tamari or coconut aminos

2 eggs

TO SERVE:

Thai basil leaves

Sliced spring onion

Lime wedges

PERUVIAN-STYLE ROAST CHICKEN WITH CORIANDER SAUCE

This South American–inspired dish is one the kids will love. The addition of paprika, cumin, honey, garlic, and chili elevates the classic roast chicken to another level. Any leftover coriander sauce is great tossed into a salad of roasted sweet potato and broccoli.

Serves: 6

3 Tbsp coconut oil or good-quality animal fat, melted

3 garlic cloves, finely chopped

3 tsp paprika

1 Tbsp ground cumin

1 Tbsp honey

Juice of 2 limes

1½ tsp sea salt

1 tsp freshly ground black pepper

1 4-lb whole chicken

2 garlic bulbs, cut in half horizontally

4 French shallots, cut into wedges

4 jalapeño chilies, cut in half lengthwise

1 cup Chicken Bone Broth (see recipe, page 87) or water

Combine the oil, chopped garlic, paprika, cumin, honey, lime juice, salt, and pepper in a large bowl and mix well. Add the chicken and rub in the marinade to evenly coat. Cover and marinate in the fridge for at least 6 hours or, for best results, overnight.

Preheat the oven to 400°F.

Transfer the chicken and any marinade in the bowl to a large casserole dish. Tie the legs together with kitchen string. Scatter the garlic bulbs, shallots, and jalapeños around the chicken, then pour in the broth.

Place in the oven and roast, basting occasionally with the juices in the dish, for 30 minutes, until the chicken is golden. Reduce the temperature to 350°F, cover with foil, and continue to cook, basting occasionally, for 45 minutes, until the chicken is cooked through.

Remove from oven and allow the chicken to rest, covered with foil, for 15 minutes.

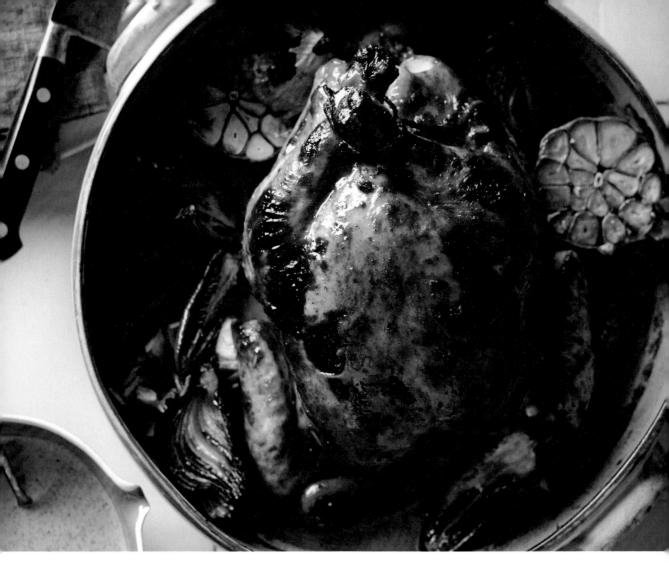

MEANWHILE, TO MAKE THE CORIANDER SAUCE, combine all the ingredients in the bowl of a food processor and blend until smooth. Season with salt and pepper.

Carve the chicken and serve with the coriander sauce and roasted vegetables.

CORIANDER SAUCE

1 jalapeño chili, seeded and roughly chopped (leave half the seeds in if you like it hot)

1 large handful coriander leaves, roughly chopped

3 garlic cloves, chopped

5 oz Mayonnaise (see recipe, page 236)

1 Tbsp lime juice

2 Tbsp extra-virgin olive oil

Sea salt and freshly ground black pepper

ROAST BEEF AND GRAVY

Roast beef is a family favorite in many homes, and rightly so. To be able to cook a nice slab of beef slowly and evenly without too much fuss is a double thumbs-up for Pete. Serve this with a big platter of roasted vegetables and you have a beautifully balanced meal.

What Pete loves about roast beef is that it tastes great cold, and when you roast an eye filet, sirloin, rib eye, chuck, or rump, there is usually a lot left over for lunches the next day. He has teamed the roast with gravy, which will keep the family happy; however, a simple salsa verde or pesto, or even some grated horseradish, is a perfect accompaniment, too.

Serves: 6 to 8

2½ lb rolled and hand-tied grass-fed roast, boneless rib eye, sirloin, or rump

2 Tbsp coconut oil or other good-quality fat

Sea salt and freshly ground black pepper

2 carrots, peeled and halved lengthwise

1 onion, skin left on, thickly sliced

1 whole garlic bulb, cloves separated and peeled

6 sprigs flat-leaf parsley

2½ cups Beef Bone Broth (see recipe, page 77)

4 sprigs thyme

Preheat the oven to 325°F.

Rub the beef with a little coconut oil and a generous pinch each of salt and pepper. Heat the oil in a large roasting pan over high heat. Add the beef and cook, turning occasionally, for 5 minutes, until well browned on all sides.

Remove the beef from the roasting pan and add the carrots, onion, garlic, and parsley sprigs in a single layer. Place the beef on top of the vegetables and add 1 cup of water. Roast for 60 minutes for medium-rare (130 to 140°F using a meat thermometer) or 65 minutes for medium (145 to 150°F). If you like your meat well done, leave it in the oven for another 10 to 15 minutes, until it reaches 155 to 165°F.

Transfer the roast beef to a carving board, cover loosely with foil, and allow it to rest for 15 minutes.

To make the gravy, discard the skin from the onion, pour in the beef broth, and place the roasting pan over medium heat. Use a wooden spoon to scrape the pan to dislodge any cooked-on bits. Add the thyme. Bring to a boil, reduce the heat to low, and simmer, stirring occasionally, for 15 minutes. Season with salt and pepper. Skim and discard the layer of fat from the surface. Place the vegetables and liquid in a blender and blend until smooth, then pass through a fine sieve. If the gravy is too thin, transfer it to a saucepan and cook over medium heat until it reaches the desired consistency.

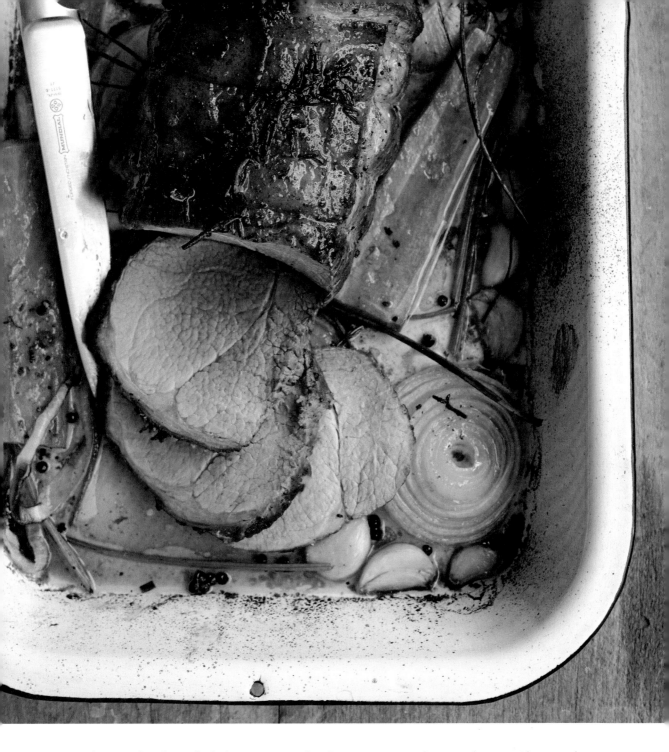

Cut the roast beef into thick slices, arrange the slices on serving plates, and serve with roasted vegetables and gravy. Leftover gravy can be transferred to an airtight container and frozen for another time. It will keep for 3 months in the freezer.

ROAST TURKEY
WITH HERB MARINADE

Pete has created a basic but delicious recipe for roasted turkey here; please feel free to play around with stuffing ingredients and accompaniments to further enhance it. You will need to start this recipe a day ahead. And if your turkey is frozen, you'll have to thaw it in the fridge for approximately 3 days first. Once thawed, leave it in the fridge until ready to cook.

Serves: 8 to 10

1 7-lb turkey

3 Tbsp duck fat, tallow, coconut oil, or other good-quality fat, melted

Sea salt and freshly ground black pepper

2 carrots, sliced lengthwise

1 onion, sliced

4 garlic cloves, peeled

5 fresh bay leaves

5 cups chicken stock (preferably homemade)

2 Tbsp tapioca flour

MARINADE

2 large handfuls mint leaves

2 large handfuls curly parsley leaves

2 large handfuls coriander leaves

4 garlic cloves, peeled

1 cup lemon juice

1 cup white wine

¾ cup duck fat, melted

2 tsp ground cumin

Sea salt and freshly ground black pepper

TO MAKE THE MARINADE, combine all the ingredients in a food processor and blend until smooth. Place the turkey in a large, shallow dish, pat dry with a paper towel, and pour over the marinade, massaging it into the skin and inside the cavity. Cover with plastic wrap and refrigerate for 24 hours. Every few hours, massage the marinade into the bird.

The next day, remove the turkey from the fridge and let it sit for 1 hour. Preheat the oven to 450°F.

TO MAKE THE STUFFING, heat the fat in a saucepan over medium heat. Add the onion and cook for 5 minutes, until soft. Crush the garlic confit and add to the pan along with the bacon. Cook until just starting to color, 3 to 5 minutes. Remove from the heat and set aside to cool. Add the remaining stuffing ingredients and mix until combined.

Fill the turkey cavity with the stuffing, cross the legs over the opening, and tie with kitchen string. Place in a large roasting pan and pour in any excess marinade. Rub the turkey with melted fat and season with salt and pepper.

Add the carrots, onion, garlic, and bay leaves, cover with foil, and place in the oven. Reduce the oven to 350°F and roast for about 2 hours and 20 minutes, basting regularly and removing the foil in the final 40 minutes to brown the skin. The turkey is done once the juices run clear when the inside of the thigh is pierced with a skewer. Cooking time may vary—it should take about 2 hours and 20 minutes. Transfer the turkey to a platter, cover with foil, and let it rest for 20 minutes.

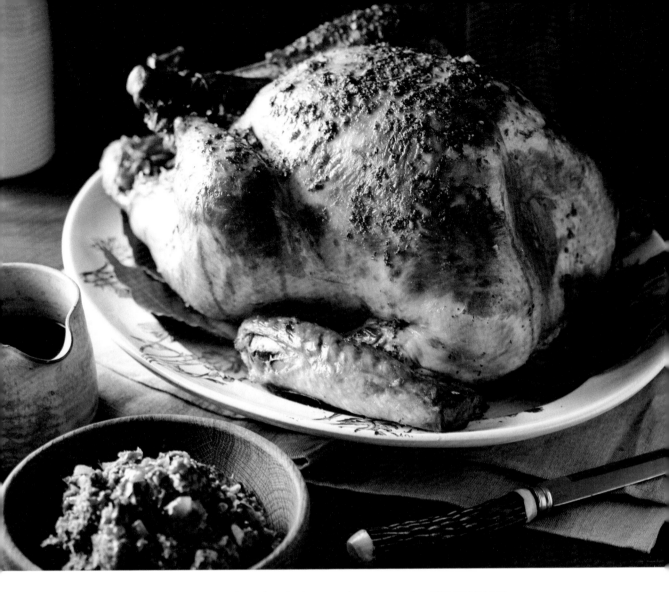

TO MAKE THE GRAVY, place the chicken stock in a saucepan over medium heat and simmer until reduced by half (about 20 minutes). Skim the fat from the roasting pan and discard. Mix the tapioca flour with 3 tablespoons of water and add to the pan. Stir in the reduced stock and bring to a boil over medium heat, stirring occasionally. Reduce the heat to low and simmer until the sauce thickens. Strain into a bowl.

Remove the stuffing from the turkey and transfer to a serving plate.

Carve the turkey and serve with the stuffing and gravy.

STUFFING

2 Tbsp duck fat, tallow, coconut oil, or other good-quality fat

1 onion, finely chopped

4 cloves garlic confit

3 rashers bacon, diced

4 Tbsp chopped curly parsley

3 Tbsp Dukkah (see recipe, page 232)

1 lb ground pork

1 tsp finely grated lemon zest

SICHUAN CHICKEN SALAD WITH EGG "NOODLES"

This Asian-inspired salad will be a hit with the kids and won't leave you with the usual heavy feeling you get after eating wheat-based noodles.

Serves: 8 to 10

1⅓ lb boneless chicken thigh fillets, skin on

2 Tbsp coconut oil, melted

Sea salt and freshly ground black pepper

1 cucumber, peeled and seeded

2 spring onions, cut into batons

1 handful coriander leaves

2 long red chilies, seeded and sliced into batons

¼ cup enoki mushrooms

½ cup Chinese cabbage, shredded

4 Tbsp bean sprouts

EGG "NOODLES"

8 eggs

Freshly ground black pepper

1½ tsp fish sauce

1 tsp tamari

4 tsp coconut oil

Coat the chicken in 2 teaspoons of the melted oil and season with salt and pepper.

Heat the remaining oil in a frying pan over medium-high heat, add the chicken, and cook for 5 minutes on each side, or until completely cooked through. Set aside and keep warm.

TO MAKE THE EGG "NOODLES," place the eggs, a little pepper, the fish sauce, and tamari in a large bowl and mix well with a fork to combine. Melt 1 teaspoon of the oil in a wok or large frying pan over medium-high heat. Pour about one-quarter of the egg mixture into the pan, swirl to form a thin layer, and cook for 30 seconds. Flip and cook for another minute, then transfer the omelet to a cutting board. Repeat this process until you have used all the egg mixture. Thinly slice the omelets into strips and set aside.

TO MAKE THE DRESSING, combine all the ingredients in a bowl with 2 tablespoons of water.

Cut the cucumber lengthwise, then scoop out and discard the seeds. Slice the cucumber into thin strips.

Place the cucumber, spring onions, coriander leaves, chilies, mushrooms, cabbage, and bean sprouts in a bowl and toss well. Add half of the dressing and toss again to combine.

Arrange the "noodles" on 4 large serving plates and top with the vegetable mixture and chicken. Spoon more dressing over the chicken and sprinkle with extra Sichuan pepper.

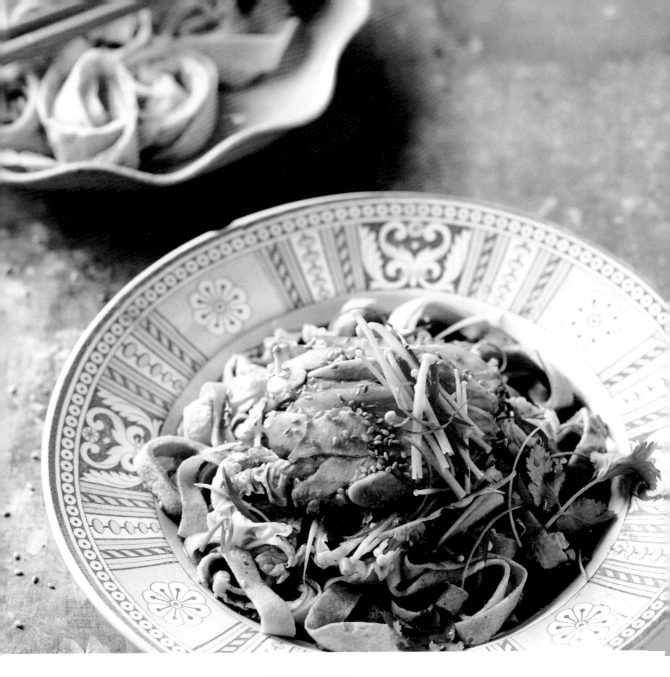

DRESSING

1 tsp finely grated ginger

1 garlic clove, crushed

2½ Tbsp tamari

1½ Tbsp sesame oil

2 Tbsp apple cider vinegar

2 Tbsp macadamia oil or extra-virgin olive oil

1 tsp coarsely ground Sichuan pepper, toasted, plus extra to serve

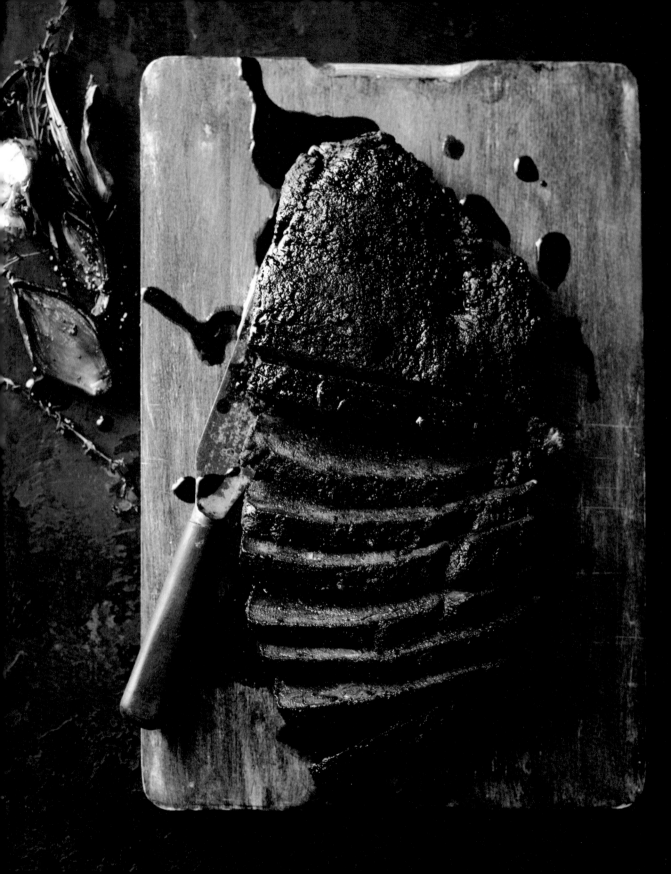

SLOW-ROASTED SPICED BRISKET

Pete guarantees the whole family will love this brisket served alongside a wonderful home-made slaw and fermented pickles or okra.

Preheat the oven to 350°F.

Mix all the spice rub ingredients together in a small bowl and set aside.

Rub the oil or fat over the brisket, then lightly season with salt and pepper. Heat a large roasting pan over high heat, add the meat, and sear on all sides for 3 to 4 minutes until browned. Then remove from the pan and transfer, fat side up, to a large plate.

When cool enough to handle, evenly coat the seared brisket with the spice rub. Arrange the shallots, garlic, and thyme in the pan in a single layer, then place the brisket on top and pour in the broth. Place the pan in the oven and roast for 20 minutes, until the spices brown.

Reduce the temperature to 300°F. Cover the brisket tightly with a damp piece of parchment paper, and tightly cover the pan with a double layer of foil. Cook in the oven for 2 hours.

Check the brisket and add ½ cup of water if the meat appears to be drying out, then tightly reseal the pan and cook for another 2 hours until the brisket is tender.

Carve the meat and serve with your choice of roasted vegetables, slaw, or fermented pickles.

Serves: 10 to 12

2 Tbsp coconut oil or good-quality animal fat, melted

4½ lb beef brisket

Sea salt and freshly ground black pepper

4 French shallots, unpeeled, cut in half lengthwise

1 garlic bulb, cut in half horizontally and broken into 8 pieces

8 thyme sprigs

1½ cups Beef Bone Broth or Chicken Bone Broth (see recipes, pages 77 and 87)

SPICE RUB

2 Tbsp smoked paprika

2 Tbsp paprika

1 Tbsp sea salt

2 tsp freshly ground black pepper

¼ tsp cayenne pepper

1 tsp ground turmeric

SPICED BEEF LIVER WITH AVOCADO SALAD

One of the joys of Pete's job is meeting the farmers and the people who produce the food that we enjoy. He was fortunate enough recently to spend a day in Tasmania at a wonderful cattle farm owned by John Bruce. While there he decided to cook heart, marrow, and liver in three separate recipes. Here is his liver recipe in all its glory. The key is to not overcook it, but keep the liver lovely and pink inside. Once you try this, it will likely become a favorite—and it is good for you, too.

Serves: 8

4 grass-fed beef liver steaks, about ⅓ lb each

2 Tbsp coconut oil or other good-quality fat

1 large handful mixed flat-leaf parsley and coriander leaves, to serve

CAJUN SPICE MIX

2 tsp sea salt

2 tsp garlic powder

2 Tbsp paprika

1 tsp freshly ground black pepper

1 tsp onion powder

1 tsp cayenne pepper

1¼ tsp dried oregano

1¼ tsp dried thyme

½ tsp chili flakes (optional)

TO MAKE THE CAJUN SPICE MIX, place all the ingredients in a bowl and combine until evenly blended.

Lightly coat the liver in 2 tablespoons of Cajun spice mix. (You can store the leftover spice mix in an airtight container in the pantry for a few months.)

Melt the oil or fat in a large frying pan over medium-high heat. Add the livers 2 at a time and cook for 1½ to 2 minutes. Flip and cook for another 1½ to 2 minutes, until still slightly pink in the middle or cooked to your liking. Allow to rest, covered in foil, for a couple of minutes.

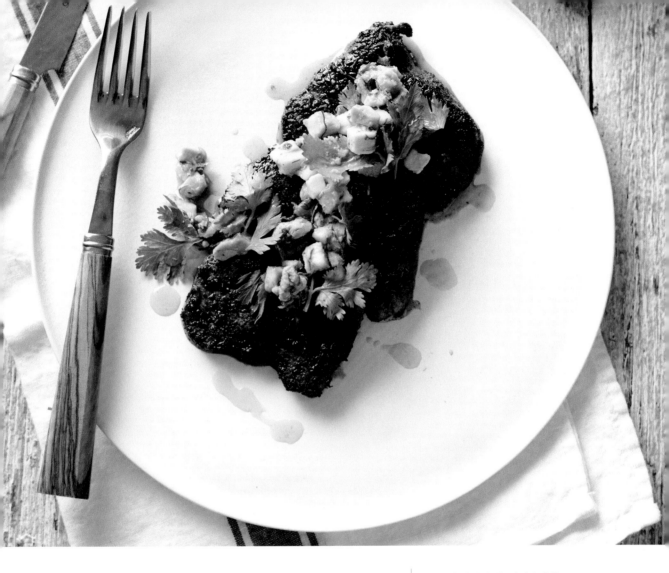

TO MAKE THE AVOCADO SALAD, place the avocados, coriander, chili, and walnuts in a bowl. In another bowl, mix the garlic, lemon juice, and olive oil to combine. Pour the dressing over the salad and gently toss. Season with salt and pepper.

Arrange the liver steaks on 4 large serving plates, top with the avocado salad, and garnish with the parsley, coriander, and extra walnuts.

AVOCADO SALAD

2 avocados, cut into ½-inch cubes

1 tsp finely chopped coriander leaves

1 long red chili, seeded and finely chopped

¼ cup activated walnuts (i.e., soaked 4 to 8 hours in salted water), toasted and crushed, plus extra to serve

1 garlic clove, finely chopped

3 Tbsp lemon juice

½ cup olive oil

Sea salt and freshly ground black pepper

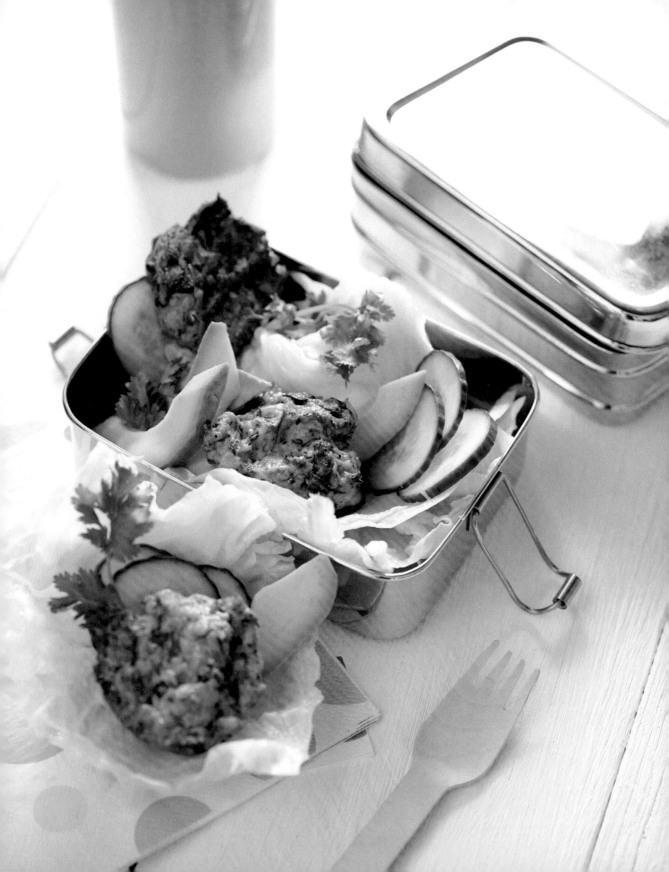

THAI CHICKEN CAKES

Pete has been lucky enough to spend some time with Michele Chevalley Hedge, who promotes a better future for coming generations by encouraging parents to cook nutrient-dense foods for their kids. Michele showed Pete a recipe that she likes to cook for her children, and it has become a family favorite in his house as well.

He has used chicken, but you could substitute turkey, fish, seafood, lamb, beef, or pretty much any other animal protein that you love. Serve these with raw or cooked vegetables and some fermented vegetables as well.

Preheat the oven to 350°F. Lightly grease an 8-cup muffin pan with coconut oil.

Place the chicken, garlic, spinach, fish sauce, turmeric, coconut cream, and ginger in a food processor and pulse a few times until finely chopped.

Spoon the chicken mixture evenly into the prepared pan. Bake for 12 minutes, until cooked through. Cool for 5 minutes before turning out. The chicken cakes will release a little bit of liquid when cooked, so drain off the liquid before you remove them from the pan.

Arrange the lettuce cups on a large platter or 4 serving plates. Place two chicken cakes inside each cup, along with some avocado, cucumber, and coriander, and squeeze over some lime juice.

Serves: 4

Coconut oil, for greasing

1 lb chicken thigh fillets, cut into pieces

2 garlic cloves, chopped

1 large handful baby spinach leaves

2 tsp fish sauce

½ tsp ground turmeric

3 Tbsp coconut cream

1 tsp finely grated ginger

TO SERVE:

4 iceberg lettuce leaves, trimmed into cups

1 avocado, sliced

½ Lebanese cucumber, peeled, seeded, and sliced

1 small handful coriander leaves

1 lime, halved

WHOLE ROASTED SALMON
WITH LEMON AND HERBS

If you can find a wild-caught Alaskan salmon and are cooking for a crowd, we recommend you prepare it as Pete has done here. There are few things that can compare with a perfectly cooked salmon perfumed with fresh herbs and lemon. Pete has teamed the salmon with a delicious salad of sweet potato and egg that is sure to make your guests extremely happy. Toss in some fermented vegetables and you will be laughing.

Serves: 6

1 small handful thyme leaves

1 small handful oregano leaves

1 lemon, thickly sliced

8 garlic cloves, halved

1½ lb whole salmon, cleaned, scaled, and gutted

Sea salt and freshly ground black pepper

2 Tbsp coconut oil or good-quality animal fat, melted

SWEET POTATO, EGG, AND WATERCRESS SALAD

2 sweet potatoes, cut into 1-inch cubes

2 Tbsp apple cider vinegar

4 Tbsp extra-virgin olive oil

1 garlic clove, crushed

Sea salt and freshly ground black pepper

2 large handfuls watercress or mesclun leaves

½ fennel bulb, very thinly sliced

3 hard-boiled eggs, peeled and crumbled

Preheat the oven to 350°F. Line a large baking pan with parchment paper and scatter one-third of the thyme, oregano, lemon, and garlic across it.

Place the fish on top of the herbs, lemon, and garlic and fill its cavity with the remaining herbs, lemon, and garlic. Season well with salt and pepper.

Drizzle the oil over the fish and roast in the oven for 50 minutes. To check if the fish is cooked, insert a metal skewer into the thickest part of the flesh. Hold the skewer there for 10 seconds, then pull it out and lightly touch it to the inside of your wrist. If the skewer feels hot, the fish is cooked. If it is only warm, cook the fish for another 10 to 15 minutes before rechecking.

TO MAKE THE SALAD, place the sweet potatoes in a saucepan of salted water and bring to a simmer. Cook until tender, about 15 minutes, then drain. Meanwhile, mix the vinegar, oil, garlic, 1 tablespoon of water, and some salt and pepper in a bowl.

Combine the sweet potato, watercress, fennel, and eggs in a large bowl, drizzle on the dressing, and lightly toss.

Serve the salmon with the salad.

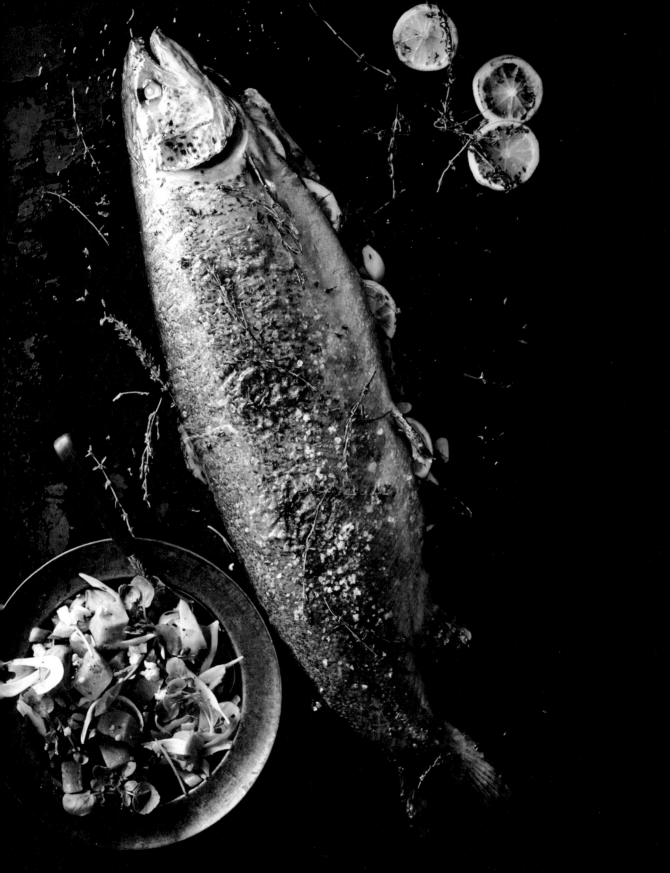

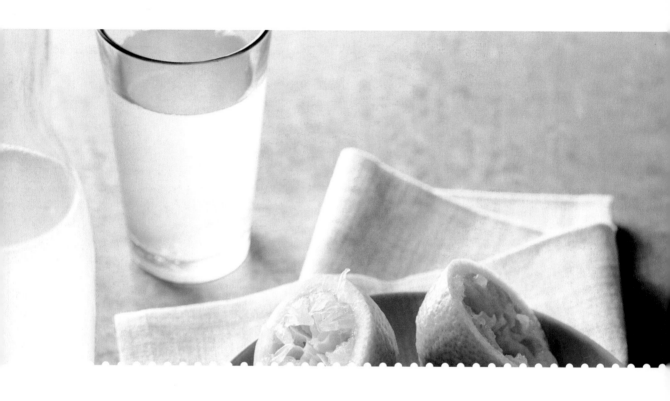

DRINKS

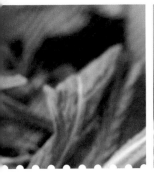
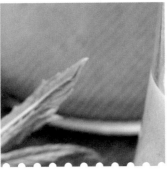
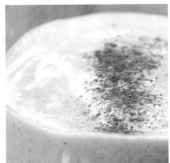
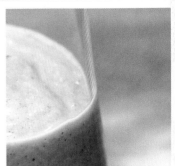

APPLE CIDER VINEGAR WATER

Having a spoonful or two of raw organic apple cider vinegar is a good habit to get into, as that little hit of tartness helps in so many ways. The ingestion of apple cider vinegar is thought to help with skin irritations, *Candida* overgrowth, acid reflux and other digestive problems, sore throats, inflamed sinuses, heart health, and blood sugar issues. A lot of people drink it to help them lose weight, but if you continue to eat the same, standard diet, then no amount of apple cider vinegar is going to help. However, the inclusion of apple cider vinegar in a low-carb high-fat diet is worth a shot (pardon the pun).

Serves: 1

2 to 3 Tbsp apple cider vinegar

4 cups warm filtered water

Stir the apple cider vinegar into the warm water and drink, on an empty stomach, within 30 minutes of waking. Food or other drinks should not be consumed for roughly 30 minutes.

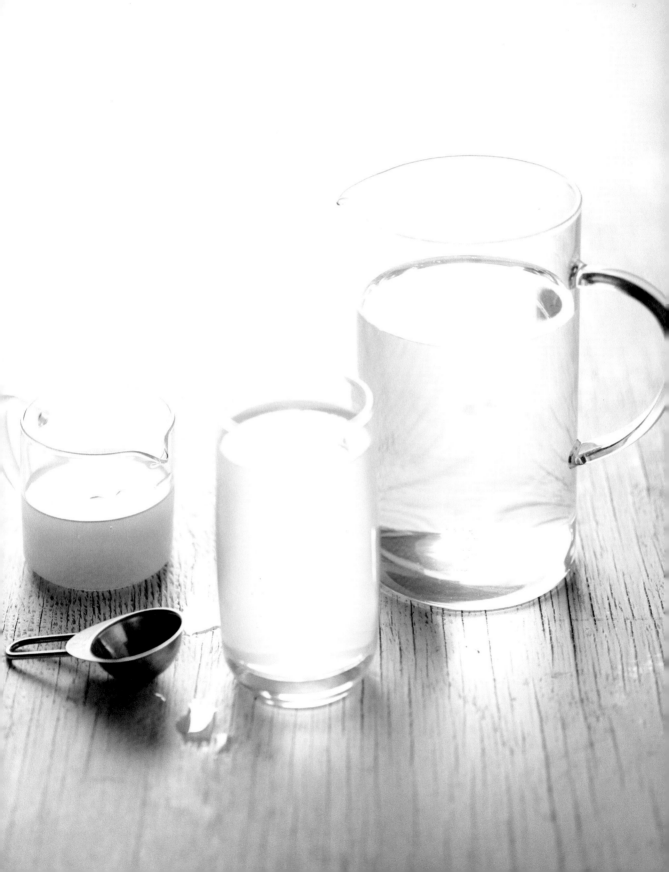

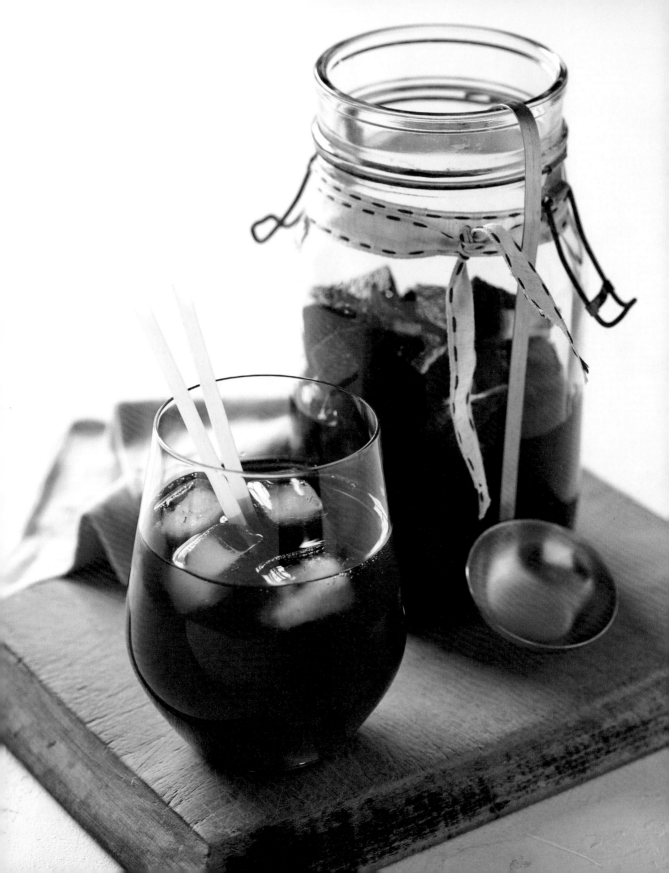

BEET KVASS

Beet kvass is an unusual and delicious drink. It is touted as a great liver cleanser and is widely used in Europe as part of a natural approach to chronic fatigue, allergies, and digestive disorders. Kvass is pretty simple to make, though you may want to wear disposable gloves to avoid staining your hands purple.

You will need a 6-cup preserving jar with an airlock lid for this recipe. Wash the jar and utensils in very hot water. Dry well and set aside. Alternatively, run them through a hot rinse cycle in the dishwasher.

Wash and peel the beets (if organic, leave the skins on). Chop the beets into small cubes, roughly ½ inch in size, and place in the jar.

Mix the salt, 1 cup of filtered water, and the sauerkraut juice or starter culture in a glass or stainless steel bowl, then pour into the jar.

Fill the jar with filtered water, leaving ¾ inch free at the top. Cover with a piece of muslin secured with an elastic band. Leave on the kitchen counter at room temperature for 3 to 5 days to ferment until the drink has reached a tanginess to your liking.

Transfer to the refrigerator and chill before drinking. The kvass will keep for 2 weeks once opened.

NOTE: If you don't want to use sauerkraut juice or starter culture, you can double the amount of salt, though this will take longer to ferment.

Makes: 6 cups

2 large beets

1 Tbsp sea salt or Himalayan salt

3 Tbsp sauerkraut juice (see recipe, page 126) or ½ packet starter culture, such as Dr. Mercola's Kinetic Culture Starter Kit for Vegetables

COCONUT AND TURMERIC KEFIR WITH GINGER AND CAYENNE

Kefir is one of the easiest fermented drinks to make, and you only have to wait 36 hours for it to ferment before bottling and popping it in the fridge. Pete likes to use young coconut water for his kefir and has added fresh turmeric and cayenne pepper to this as it is a natural anti-inflammatory and powerful antioxidant. If you are sensitive to chilies, just leave out the cayenne.

Serves: 4

3 young coconuts

2 probiotic capsules or 2 to 3 Tbsp water kefir grains

1½ Tbsp finely grated fresh turmeric or 1½ tsp ground turmeric

1½ Tbsp finely grated ginger

Pinch of cayenne pepper (or more if desired)

You will need a 1-quart glass jar for this recipe. Wash the jar and a nonmetal spoon in hot, soapy water, then run them through the dishwasher on a hot rinse cycle to sterilize. Alternatively, place the jar and spoon in a large saucepan filled with water and boil for 10 minutes. Put on a baking tray in a 300°F oven to dry.

Open the coconuts by cutting off the tops. Strain the coconut water into the sterilized jar. If using a probiotic capsule, open up the capsule. Add the probiotic powder or water kefir grains to the coconut water, then add the turmeric, ginger, and cayenne. Stir well with the sterilized spoon. Cover with a piece of muslin and a rubber band. Place in the pantry or in a dark spot for 24 to 48 hours to ferment.

Taste-test the kefir after 24 to 30 hours. Pour some into a glass—it should taste sour, with no sweetness left, like coconut beer. (Some batches are fizzier than others, but all are beneficial.) If it still tastes sweet, place it back in the pantry for the remaining recommended fermentation time. When you're happy with the flavor, pour through a sieve to remove the water kefir grains (if using) and return the kefir to the jar. Keep in the fridge for up to 2 months. The water kefir grains can be stored in coconut water in the fridge until you make your next batch (refresh the coconut water every 5 days or so).

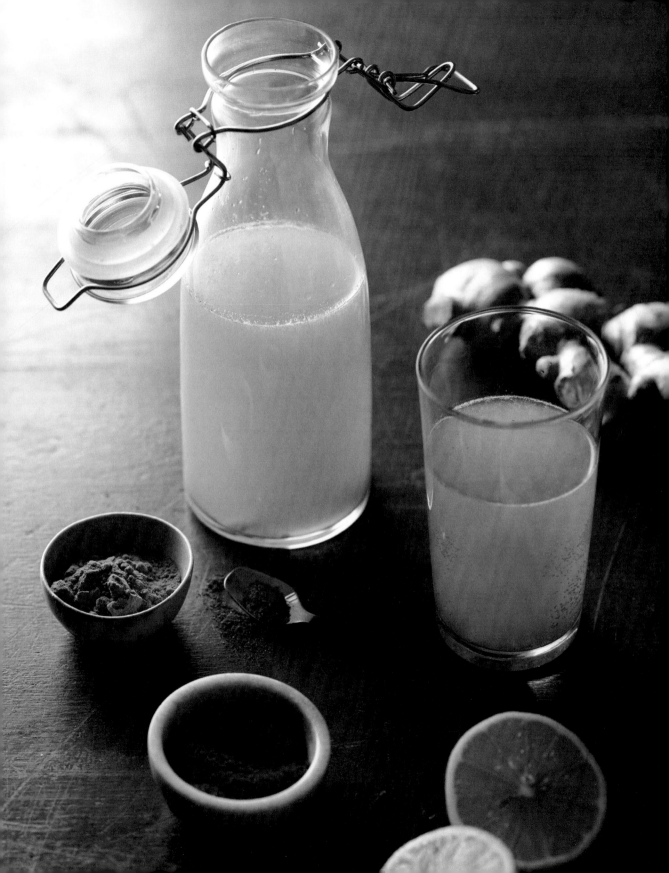

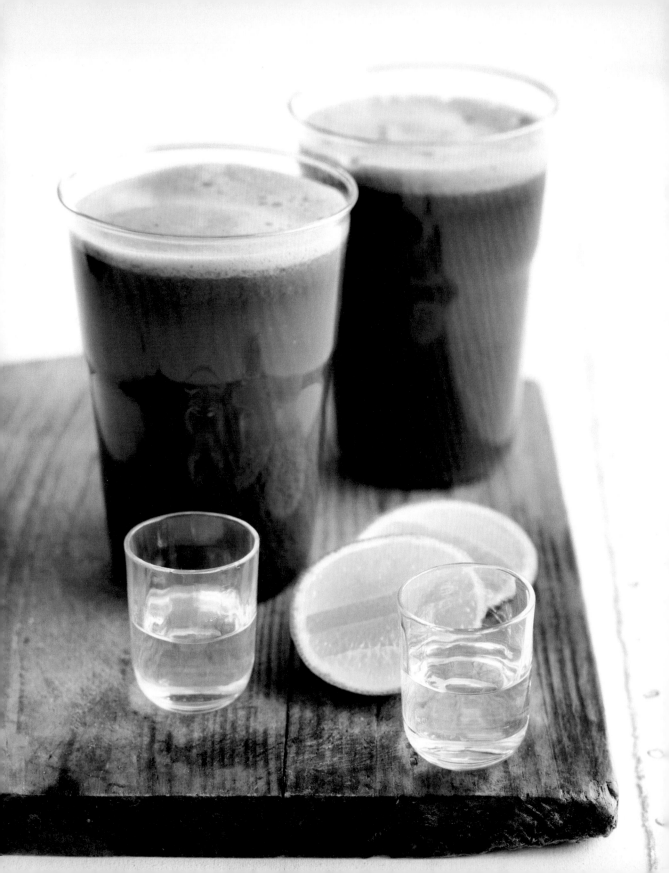

GREEN JUICE WITH OIL

If you feel like having a green juice, we strongly urge you to add a shot of MCT oil. Now, a lot of green juices you can buy are full of fruit, which is a sugar bomb, so we have included a low-sugar version for you here, as we know some people love to have juice daily. Just remember to go easy on the sweet fruit. For more information on MCT oil, see page 209.

Juice the spinach, apples, mint, parsley, cucumber, lime, and ginger. Add the oil and stir well.

Pour the juice into glasses and serve with ice, if desired.

NOTE: MCT oil can be found in health food stores or online.

Serves: 2 to 4

¼ cup English spinach, trimmed (optional substitutes include baby spinach, kale, and Swiss chard)

2 green apples, cored

1 small handful mint leaves and stalks

1 small handful flat-leaf parsley

1 cucumber, peeled and seeded

1 lime, peeled and chopped

1½ inch piece of ginger, peeled and chopped

2 Tbsp coconut oil, melted, or 2 Tbsp MCT oil (see note)

Ice cubes (optional)

GREEN SMOOTHIE

Avocados, coconuts, nuts, seeds, and eggs are just some of the wonderful sources of the healthy fats that our bodies need to thrive. Try having one of these bad boys (or should we say good guys) for breakfast one day a week and just see how you feel for the next 3 to 4 hours. Try different herbs and spices and see what you like most. You can also try freezing any leftover smoothie mix in frozen pop molds for a treat on a hot day—the kids will love it!

Serves: 2 to 4

2 young coconuts (flesh and water) or 2 cups coconut water

1 ripe avocado, pit and skin removed

1½ oz Swiss chard, spinach, or kale, roughly chopped

1 large handful fresh mint leaves, parsley, or coriander

1 free-range organic egg

8 walnuts, soaked in water overnight

8 macadamia nuts, soaked in water overnight

½ tsp ground cinnamon

Seeds of 1 split vanilla pod or ½ tsp vanilla extract

Filtered water, nut milk, or coconut milk, added to reach desired consistency

Chop a square opening in the top of each coconut (preferably with 4 incisions made with a cleaver) and pour the coconut water directly into a blender container. Scrape out the soft coconut flesh from the inside of the coconut shell with a spoon and chop the flesh into chunks.

Drain and rinse the soaking walnuts and macadamias.

Add the coconut flesh and all other ingredients except the filtered water into the blender and blend until smooth. Add filtered water slowly until you reach the desired consistency. Serve immediately, either in tall milkshake glasses or in coconut shells with a straw.

NOTE: You can presoak the nuts and store them in an airtight container in the fridge for up to 4 days.

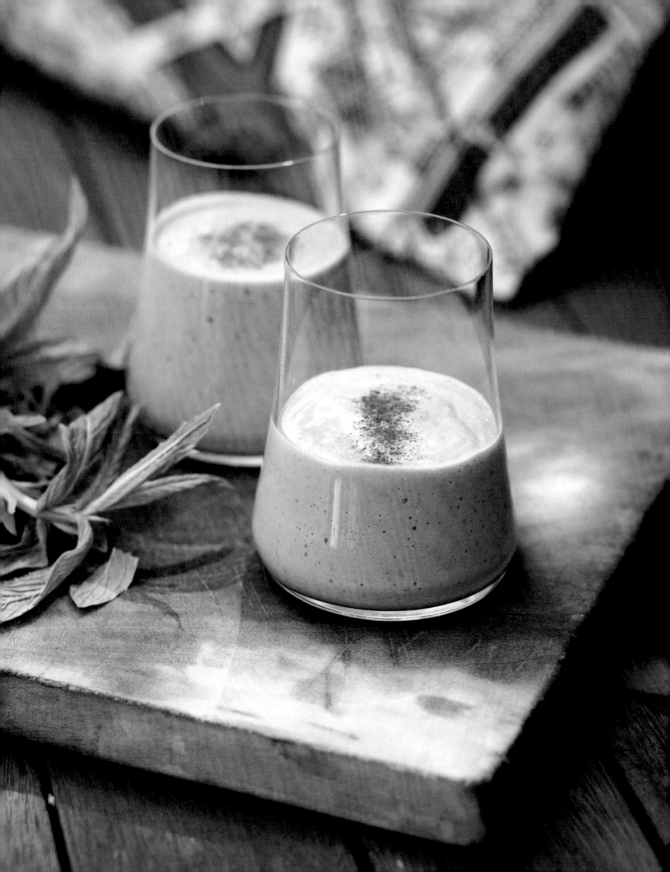

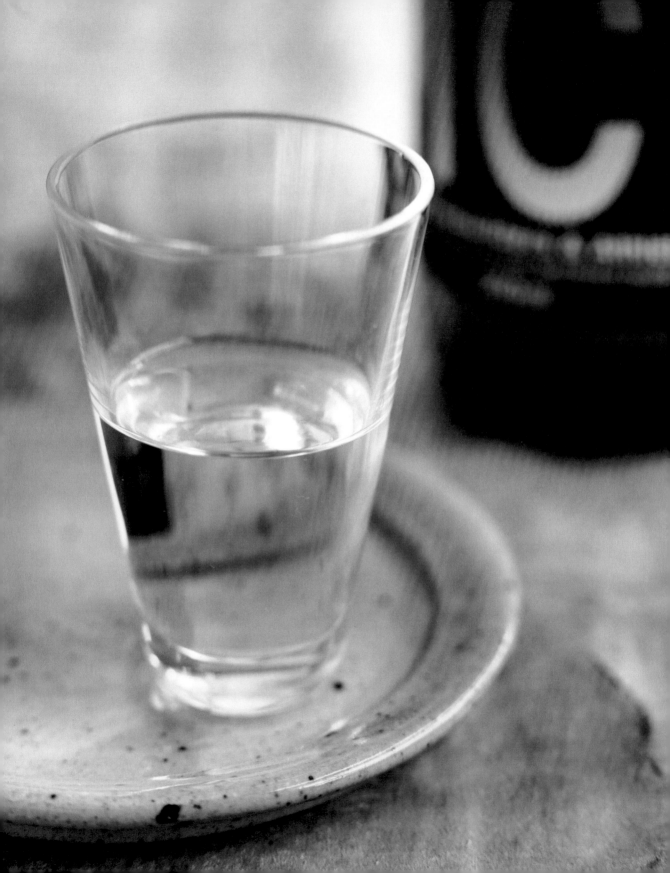

MCT OIL

MCT stands for medium-chain triglycerides, a special type of saturated fatty acid that is easily digested to provide fast, sustained energy. While this isn't a recipe per se, we've included it in Drinks because it contains a plethora of benefits. For starters, MCT oil is believed to improve cognitive function and help maintain a healthy body weight. It's also great for balancing hormones, regulating blood sugar, and supporting gut health, and it has antibacterial and antifungal properties.

Take 1 teaspoon to 1 tablespoon per day. To start, take 1 teaspoon; then, over the course of a few weeks, gradually add ½ teaspoon every week or so. MCT oil on an empty stomach can cause nausea, so it's best to have it with food. If you are experiencing GI distress or diarrhea, cut the dosage back.

MCT oil (can be found in health food stores or online)

SUNSHINE MILK

Having a cup of the delicious ancient Ayurvedic drink golden milk every day is a nourishing way to add more of the wonder spice turmeric to your diet. Turmeric's many healing benefits and vibrant golden color come from its key active ingredient, curcumin, a powerful antioxidant and anti-inflammatory. You can enjoy this hot in the cooler months and chilled or frozen when it's warmer. In the recipe for Macadamia Milk below, we strain out the nuts; however, you can also blend them into the milk to make a thicker and creamier drink.

Serves: 2

1½ tsp coconut oil

5 cardamom pods, crushed

1 tsp Turmeric Paste (see below)

2 cups Macadamia Milk (see recipe below) or coconut milk or almond milk

Pinch freshly ground black pepper

½ tsp vanilla extract

1 tsp honey or maple syrup (optional)

Ground cinnamon, to serve

TURMERIC PASTE

4 Tbsp ground turmeric

1 cup water

MACADAMIA MILK

1 cup macadamia nuts

Place the coconut oil and cardamom in a saucepan and cook over medium-high heat until fragrant, about 1 minute. Reduce the heat to medium, add the remaining ingredients except the cinnamon, and stir for a few minutes until warmed through. Strain through a fine sieve. Pour into glasses or mugs and enjoy with a sprinkle of cinnamon on top.

TO MAKE THE TURMERIC PASTE, place the turmeric and the water in a small saucepan. Simmer over low heat, stirring occasionally, until you have a creamy and smooth paste, about 15 minutes.

NOTE: The leftover turmeric paste will keep for 2 to 3 weeks stored in an airtight glass container in the fridge.

FOR THE MACADAMIA MILK, place the macadamia nuts in a bowl, cover with 1 liter of filtered water, and soak for 8 hours or overnight. Drain and rinse well. Place the nuts in a high-powered blender with 1 liter of filtered water and blend until smooth. Line a bowl with a piece of muslin so that the muslin hangs over the edges of the bowl (alternatively, you can use a nut milk bag). Pick up the edges of the muslin, bring together, and twist to squeeze out all of the milk. (The leftover solids can be used to make bliss balls—that's a term for a bite-sized morsel packed with minerals, vitamins, and benefits—or used in place of

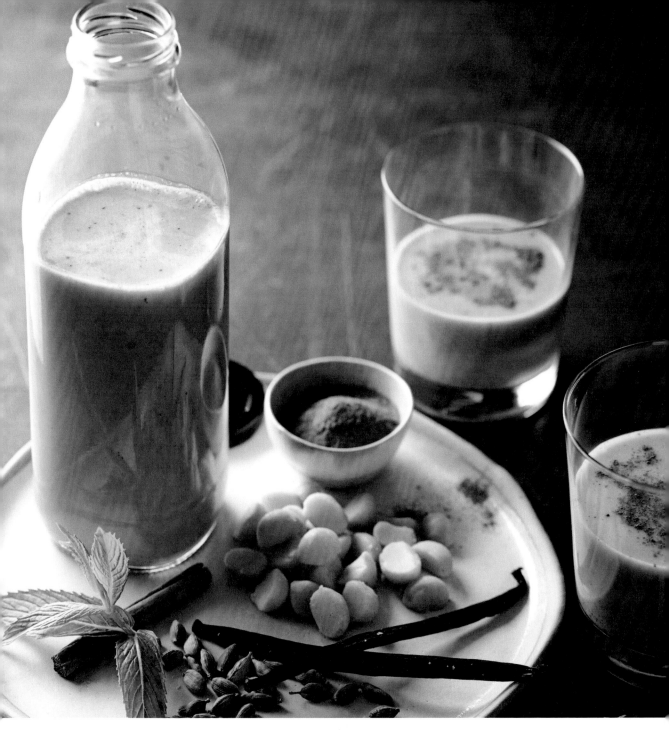

almond meal in baking recipes.) Pour the nut milk into a sterilized 1-liter bottle or jar, then refrigerate until ready to use. Shake the bottle before use as the milk will settle and separate after time.

NOTE: The leftover nut milk will keep in the fridge for 3 to 4 days.

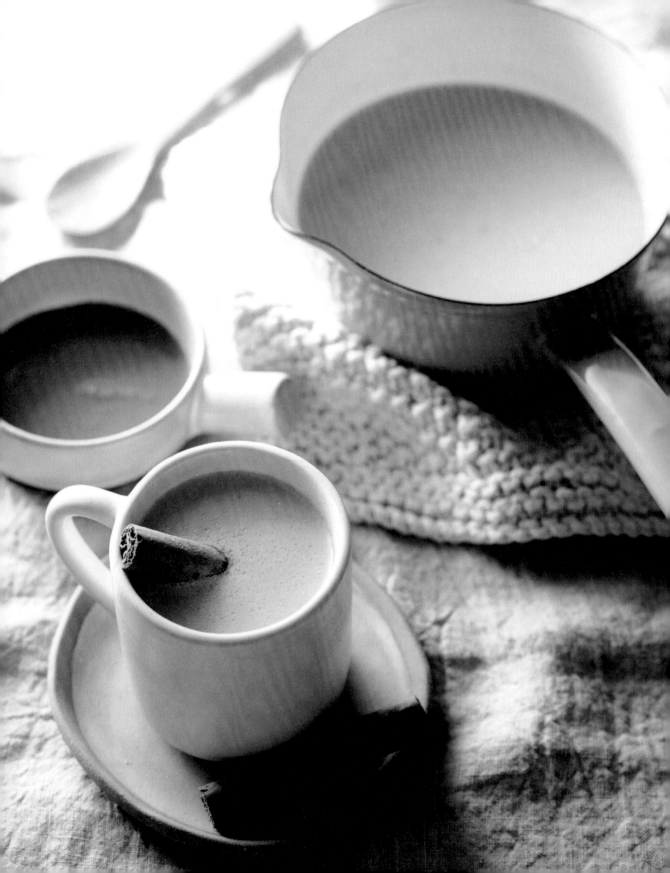

TURMERIC LATTE

Add 2 cups almond milk, 1 teaspoon turmeric paste, ground cinnamon, pepper, and honey (if using) to a saucepan over medium-low heat and stir for a few minutes until warmed through. Strain through a fine sieve over a jug.

Pour into 2 mugs and enjoy with a cinnamon stick to sip the warm turmeric latte. (The leftover nut milk will keep in the fridge for 3 to 4 days; the leftover turmeric paste will keep for 2 to 3 weeks stored in an airtight glass container in the fridge.)

FOR THE TURMERIC PASTE, place the turmeric and the water in a small saucepan. Simmer over low heat, stirring occasionally, until you have a creamy and smooth paste, about 15 minutes.

TO MAKE THE ALMOND MILK, place the almonds in a bowl, cover with 4 cups of the filtered water, and soak for 8 hours or overnight. Drain and rinse well. Place the nuts in a high-powered blender with the remaining 4 cups of filtered water and blend until smooth. Line a bowl with a piece of muslin so that the muslin hangs over the edges of the bowl (alternatively, you can use a nut milk bag). Pick up the edges of the muslin, bring together, and twist to squeeze out all of the milk. (The leftover solids can be used to make bliss balls—bite-sized morsels packed with minerals, vitamins, and benefits—or used in place of almond meal in baking recipes.) Pour the nut milk into a sterilized 1-quart bottle or jar and refrigerate until ready to use. Shake the bottle before use as the milk will settle and separate over time.

Serves: 2

2 cups Almond Milk (see below) or coconut milk

1 tsp Turmeric Paste (see below)

½ tsp ground cinnamon

1 pinch freshly ground black pepper

1 tsp honey or maple syrup (optional)

Cinnamon sticks, to serve

TURMERIC PASTE

4 Tbsp ground turmeric

1 cup water

ALMOND MILK

1 cup skinless almonds

8 cups filtered water

TURMERIC, LEMON, AND GINGER JUICE WITH OIL

This could become one of your favorite drinks of all time. The mixture of lemon, turmeric, and ginger with a hint of coconut or MCT oil makes for a very powerful and potent medicinal drink. You can prepare this a couple of ways: either pop the lemon flesh, turmeric, and ginger in a juicer or hand-squeeze the lemon and blitz everything else in a blender. If you find the lemon a little strong, you can use grapefruit or orange juice instead.

Serves: 2

2 cups coconut water

2-inch piece fresh turmeric or 1 tsp ground turmeric

1-inch piece ginger, sliced

1 Tbsp coconut oil or MCT oil

Juice of ½ lemon

½ tsp sea salt (optional)

Place the coconut water, turmeric, ginger, and coconut oil in a blender and blend until smooth. Strain into a jug (discard the leftover ginger and turmeric pulp). Stir in the lemon juice and the salt (if using), pour into glasses, and serve.

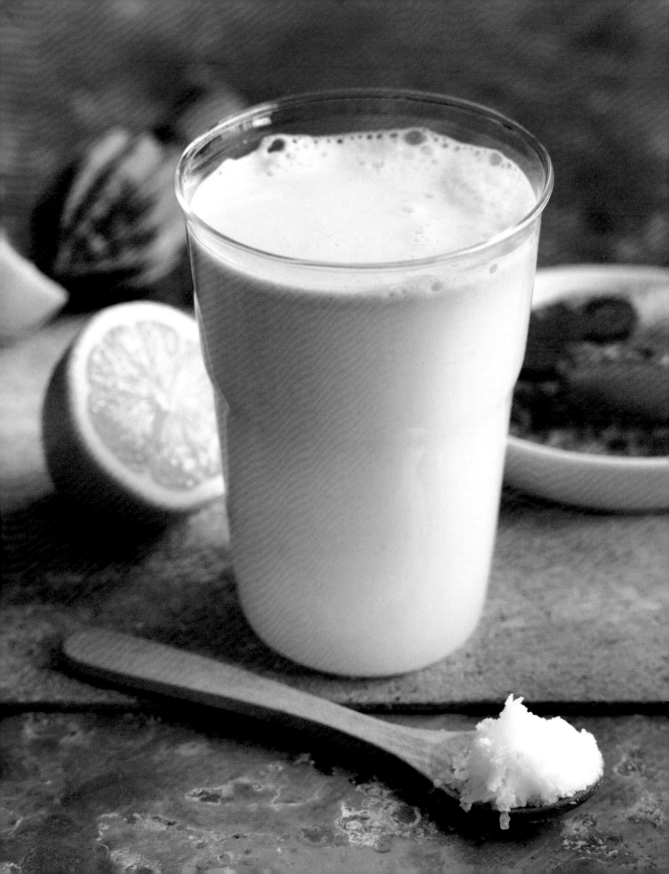

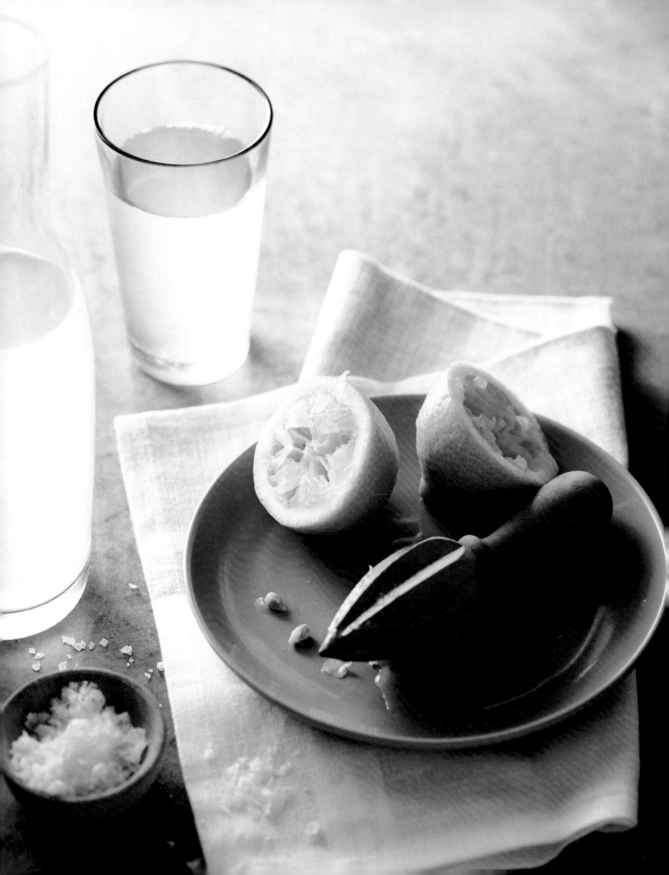

WATER WITH
LEMON AND SALT

This is another drink you may wish to add to your daily or weekly routine, or alternate with the Apple Cider Vinegar Water on page 198. Lemon and good-quality salt like Himalayan or sea salt in filtered water can help fight inflammation and add much-needed trace minerals. This combination also boosts your immune system through the addition of vitamin C and can help you detox as well. This amazing little drink is great for skin, helps with sleep issues, and is wonderful for blood sugar levels.

Combine all ingredients and stir until the salt has dissolved. Drink on an empty stomach within 30 minutes of waking. Food or other drinks should not be consumed for 30 minutes.

Serves: 1

4 cups warm filtered water

2 Tbsp lemon juice

2 tsp sea salt

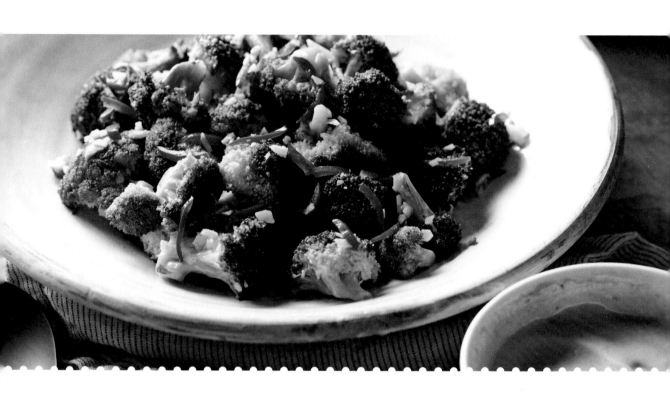

SIDES AND CONDIMENTS

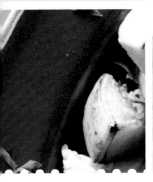
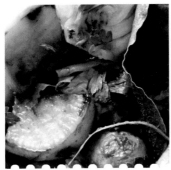
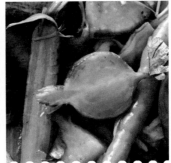
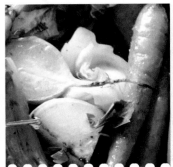

ASIAN SLAW

This recipe is great served with a grilled, steamed, or poached piece of meat or with a few spoonfuls of fermented vegetables. You can change the dressing to make this slaw match any cuisine: use tahini for a Middle Eastern dish, chimichurri to make it South American, or nam jim for a Southeast Asian feel. Or to create a classic coleslaw, simply use homemade mayonnaise and dill.

Serves: 6 as a side dish

3 cups shredded Chinese cabbage (wong bok)

3 cups shredded red cabbage

1 large carrot, julienned

5 large radishes, julienned

4 spring onions, white and green parts, finely sliced

1 to 2 long red chilies, seeded and julienned

1 red bell pepper, seeded and julienned

1 to 2 large handfuls coriander leaves

1 cup bean sprouts

Sea salt and freshly ground black pepper

ASIAN DRESSING

3 Tbsp miso paste or tahini

1 Tbsp tamari or coconut aminos

2 tsp finely grated ginger

1 garlic clove, finely chopped

2 Tbsp apple cider vinegar

1 Tbsp Mayonnaise (see recipe, page 236)

1 Tbsp lemon juice or yuzu juice

1 tsp honey (optional)

3 Tbsp avocado oil or olive oil

2 Tbsp sesame oil

TO MAKE THE DRESSING, in a small bowl, whisk together the miso, tamari, ginger, garlic, vinegar, mayonnaise, lemon juice, and honey (if using). Slowly whisk in the avocado oil and sesame oil until emulsified. Set aside.

TO MAKE THE SLAW, combine all the ingredients in a large bowl, add half of the dressing, and toss gently. Add a little more dressing if desired, then store any remaining dressing in a sealed glass jar in the fridge (use within 3 to 4 days).

Check the seasoning and add more salt and pepper if needed.

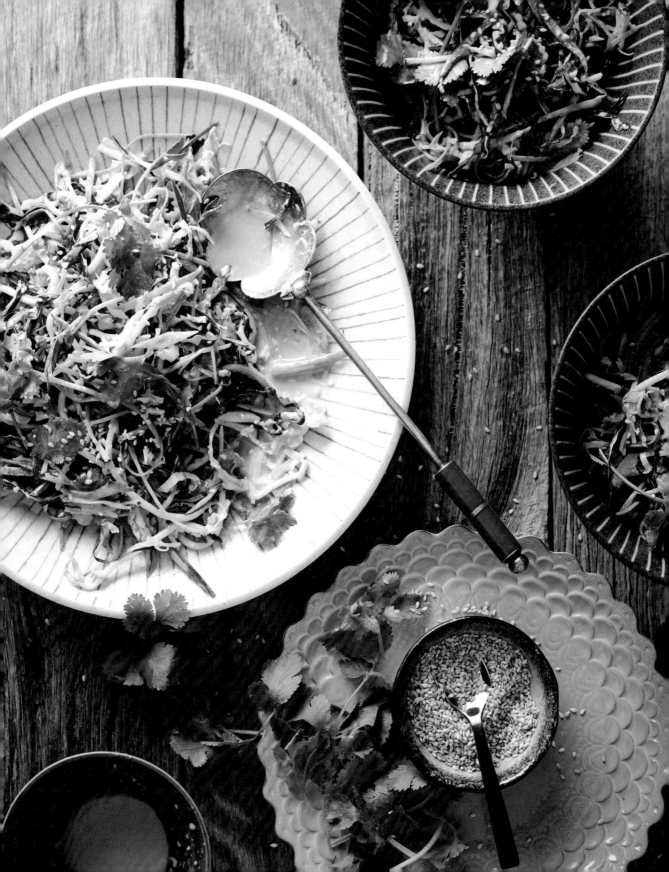

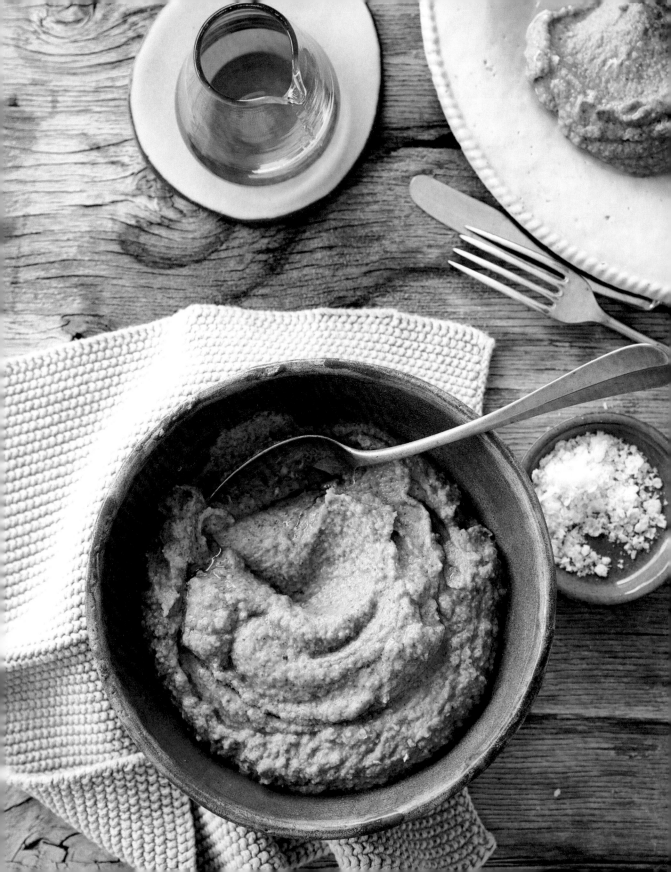

BROCCOLI MASH

Broccoli doesn't just taste good; it's been proven over and over to contain amazing compounds that are packed with nutrition. This mouthwatering Broccoli Mash recipe is no exception. Give it a try today!

Fill a saucepan with water and place a steamer with a lid on top. Bring to a boil. Place the broccoli florets in the steamer, cover, and steam for 30 minutes, until the broccoli is very soft. Place the broccoli in the bowl of a food processor and process until smooth. Add the coconut oil and blitz again, then season to taste with salt and pepper.

Transfer the broccoli mash to a serving bowl and drizzle some extra-virgin olive oil over the top.

Serves: 2 to 4

2 large heads broccoli, chopped into florets

2 Tbsp coconut oil or good-quality animal fat, melted

1 Tbsp extra-virgin olive oil, to serve

Sea salt and freshly ground black pepper

BROCCOLI "RICE"

Broccoli is a nutritional powerhouse that is often featured on Pete's family table. It provides your body with dozens, maybe even hundreds, of super-nutrients that support optimal, body-wide health. That makes this flavorsome "rice" a quick, convenient, and most importantly, healthy dish to serve with your next meal.

Serves: 4

2 heads organic broccoli, 7 oz each, roughly chopped

2 Tbsp coconut oil

Sea salt and freshly ground black pepper

Place the broccoli in the bowl of a food processor and pulse into tiny pieces the size of grains of rice.

In a frying pan, heat the coconut oil over medium heat, add the broccoli "rice," and lightly cook for 4 to 6 minutes, until softened. Season with salt and pepper and serve.

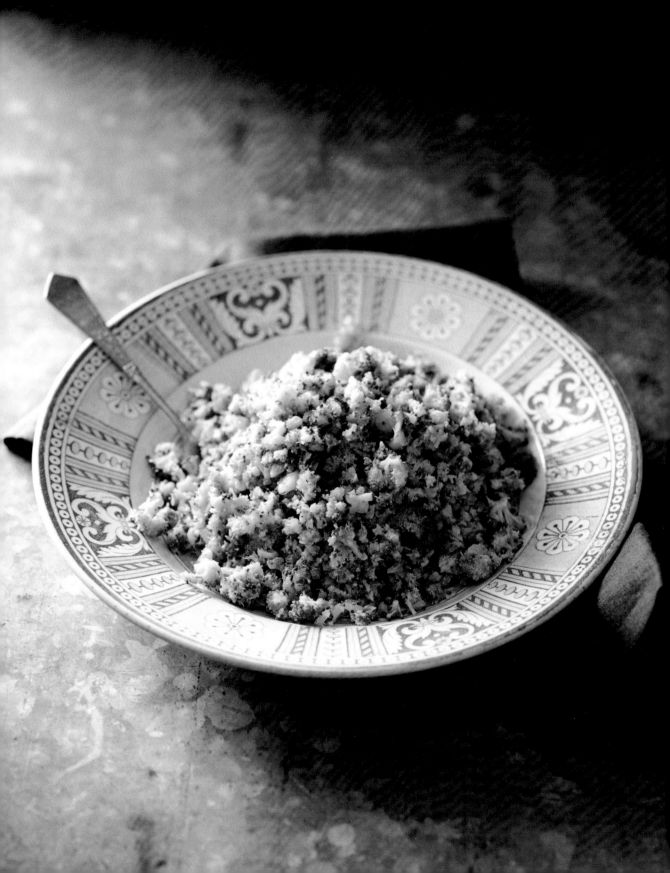

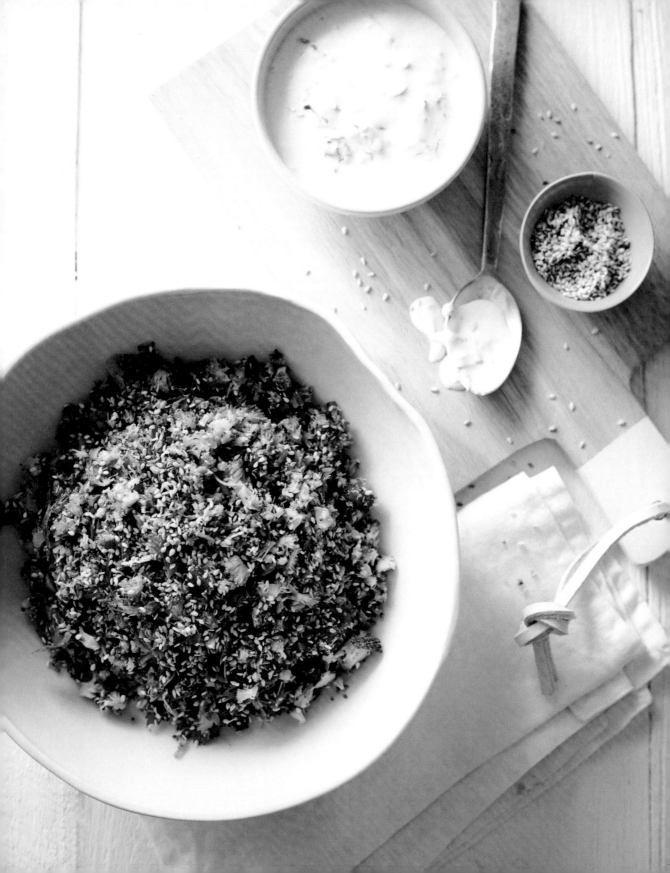

BROCCOLI TABBOULEH

Pete enjoys giving classic recipes a creative twist and wondered how he could jazz up broccoli, enhance its flavor, and take it to another level. Then one day when he was looking at some tabbouleh, he thought, why not mix finely chopped broccoli into this delicious salad? Success! Pete has used raw broccoli here, but you could easily blanch or roast yours. This is a perfect accompaniment to grilled seafood or roast lamb or chicken.

Place the broccoli in a food processor bowl and pulse until it resembles rice, then transfer to a large bowl. Stir in the tomatoes, parsley, red onion, spring onion, and chia seeds and set aside.

TO MAKE THE DRESSING, use a mortar and pestle to pound the garlic with a pinch of salt to form a thick paste. Add the lemon juice and olive oil and mix until well combined.

Add the dressing to the broccoli mixture and season with salt and pepper. Mix gently, then allow to stand for 10 minutes so the flavors can develop.

Place the tabbouleh in a large bowl and serve.

Serves: 4

1½ heads broccoli, cut into florets (reserve the stems for making stock)

4 tomatoes, seeded and diced

2 large handfuls flat-leaf parsley, chopped

½ red onion, diced

2 spring onions, finely sliced

2 Tbsp chia seeds (soaked)

Sea salt and freshly ground black pepper

DRESSING

2 garlic cloves, peeled

Sea salt

4 Tbsp lemon juice

½ cup extra-virgin olive oil

BROCCOMOLE

Ha ha! You have to have a laugh when it comes to making up dish titles. Here is the wonderful broccomole, which takes its name from mixing the classic guacamole with broccoli. Pete prefers to use cooked and chilled broccoli in the mix, but you can use raw broccoli if you choose.

For something a little fun, you can also add some cooked or raw fish and try it as a filling for nori rolls. Feel free to add toasted seeds for a little more flavor and texture.

Serves: 2

½ cup broccoli florets

1 avocado, diced or mashed

1 garlic clove, finely diced

1 Tbsp lemon juice

½ tsp chili flakes (optional)

1 Tbsp extra-virgin olive oil

Sea salt and freshly ground black pepper

TO SERVE:

Lemon wedges

Seed crackers or sweet potato crisps (optional)

Bring a saucepan of salted water to a boil. Add broccoli and cook for 3 minutes, until just tender. Drain, then plunge the broccoli into ice-cold water to stop the cooking process. When the broccoli is completely cold, drain again and shake off any excess water. Chop the cooled broccoli into small pieces and set aside.

Place the avocado, garlic, lemon juice, chili flakes (if using), oil, and broccoli in a serving bowl and mix well. Season with salt and pepper. Serve with lemon wedges and some seed crackers or sweet potato crisps, if desired.

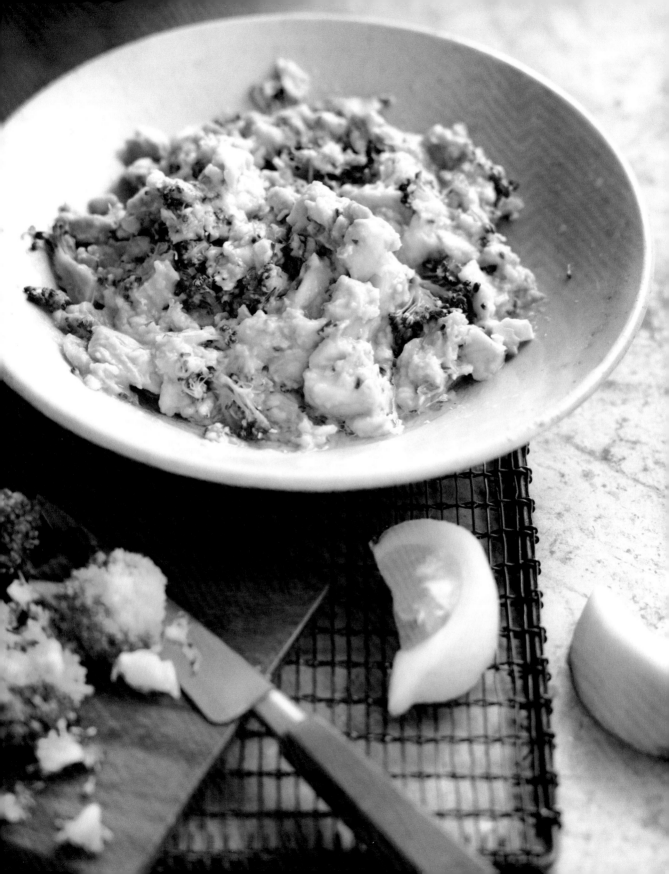

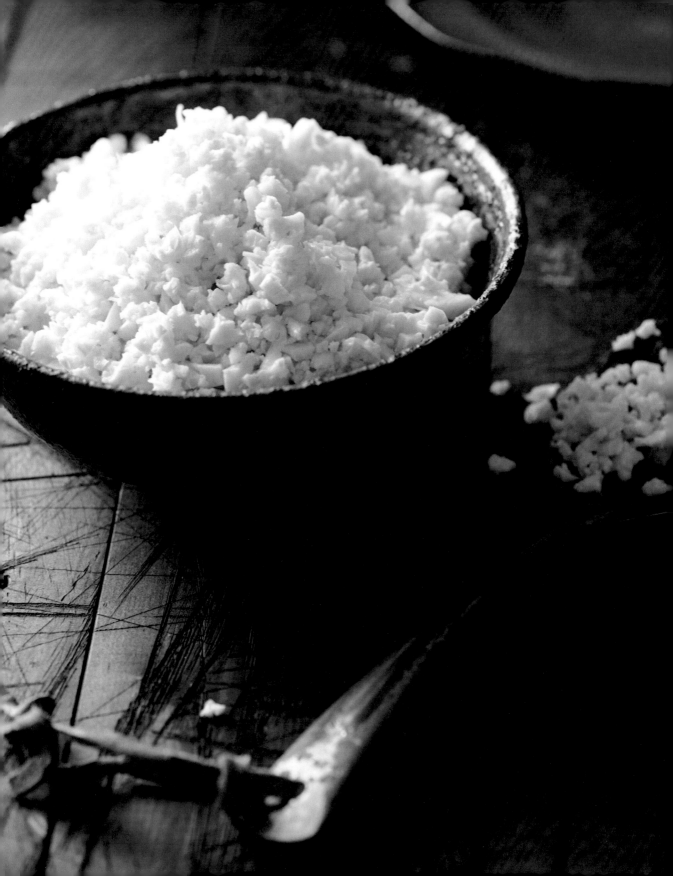

CHILI OIL

Heat the oil in a saucepan over low heat. Add the chili flakes and warm for 2 minutes. Do not boil. Remove from the heat and cool.

Store in a sealed glass jar or bottle in a cool, dark place. Shake the bottle every week or so. The longer you leave it, the hotter and redder the oil becomes.

Makes: Approximately 2 cups

1¾ cups olive oil

4 Tbsp chili flakes

COCONUT CAULIFLOWER RICE

Place the cauliflower in the bowl of a food processor and pulse into tiny, fine pieces that resemble rice.

Heat the oil in a large pan over medium heat. Add the onion and cook for 5 minutes, until softened and translucent. Add the spices (if using) and stir until fragrant, about 10 seconds.

Add the cauliflower rice, coconut milk, and broth to the pan, stir to combine, and simmer, stirring occasionally, for 8 to 10 minutes, until the cauliflower rice is cooked through and has thickened slightly. Season with salt and pepper and serve sprinkled with the coriander and mint.

Serves: 4 to 6

1 head organic cauliflower, roughly chopped

1 Tbsp coconut oil

½ onion, finely chopped

½ tsp ground cardamom (optional)

½ tsp ground cumin (optional)

One 13-oz can coconut milk

½ cup Chicken Bone Broth (see recipe, page 87) or water

Sea salt and freshly ground black pepper

Coriander and mint leaves, to serve

DUKKAH

Makes: About 2 cups

½ cup pine nuts

⅓ cup soaked coriander seeds

½ tsp ground cumin

½ tsp sea salt

½ tsp chili powder

½ tsp baharat

Pinch of dried mint

Combine the pine nuts and soaked coriander seeds in a large dry frying pan and toast over medium-high heat for 1 minute, or until the mix has started to color.

Pour the nut and seed mix into a food processor. Add the cumin, salt, chili powder, baharat, and mint and pulse to combine.

Use the dukkah as a seasoning in cooking or serve with sprouted seed bread, cashew cheese, and extra-virgin olive oil. Store in an airtight container in the pantry for 2 to 3 weeks.

OLIVE TAPENADE

This zesty, tasty mixture is sure to leave your taste buds watering for more.

Makes: About ¾ cup

½ cup pitted black or green olives

Juice and zest of ½ lemon

8 basil leaves

2 garlic cloves, peeled

2 salted anchovy fillets, rinsed and patted dry

10 salted baby capers, rinsed well and patted dry

3 Tbsp olive oil

Put everything except the oil into a food processor bowl and process until well combined. With the motor running, drizzle in the oil and process until the mixture reaches a nice, thick paste consistency. Store in a glass jar in the fridge for up to 2 weeks.

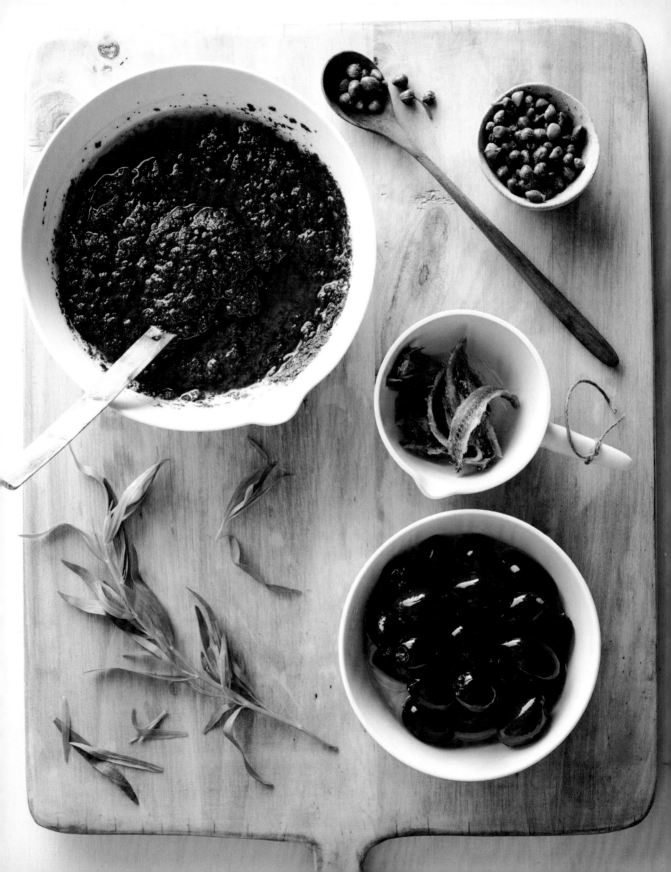

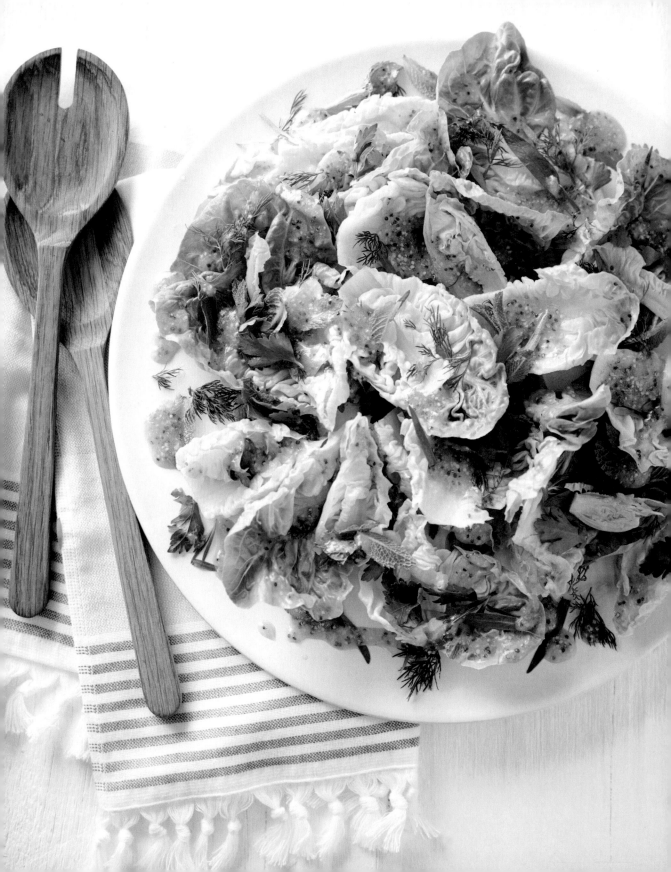

FRESH ROMAINE SALAD WITH MUSTARD VINAIGRETTE

"Less is more" has always been and will always be a chef's mantra. This entails letting the ingredients shine as much as possible. Sure, there are amazing recipes—such as curries—that include 20 ingredients, but the underlying factor in these complex dishes is that everything is in balance without one flavor dominating another.

And then we have dishes like this one, which is really just some awesome, crunchy, pristine leaves lightly coated with a playful dressing that brings everything to life. Pete encourages you to play around with different dressings and vinaigrettes and become a master salad maker at home.

Tear the romaine leaves into smaller pieces.

Combine the herbs and romaine in a serving bowl. Drizzle on the mustard vinaigrette and add a little salt and pepper, if you like. Serve immediately.

FOR THE MUSTARD VINAIGRETTE, combine all the ingredients in a screw-top jar. Screw the lid on firmly and shake well. Store in the fridge for up to 5 days. Shake well before using.

Serves: 4

4 baby romaine lettuces, leaves separated

2 handfuls mixed herbs (such as tarragon, dill, mint, flat-leaf parsley, and basil leaves)

⅓ cup Mustard Vinaigrette (see recipe below)

Sea salt and freshly ground black pepper

MUSTARD VINAIGRETTE

Makes: 1½ cups

4 Tbsp apple cider vinegar or lemon juice

2 Tbsp whole-grain mustard

1 tsp sea salt

¼ tsp freshly ground black pepper

1 garlic clove, finely chopped

1 cup extra-virgin olive oil or macadamia oil

MAYONNAISE

Makes: 1 lb

4 egg yolks

2 tsp Dijon mustard

1 Tbsp apple cider vinegar

1 Tbsp lemon juice

1½ cup olive oil or macadamia oil, or ¾ cup of each

Sea salt and freshly ground black pepper

Place the egg yolks, mustard, vinegar, lemon juice, oil, and a pinch of salt in a glass jug or jar.

Blend with a handheld blender until smooth and creamy. Season with salt and pepper. Store in a sealed glass jar in the fridge for 4 to 5 days.

TIP: Alternatively, you can place the egg yolks, mustard, vinegar, lemon juice, and a pinch of salt in the bowl of a food processor and process until combined. With the motor running, slowly pour in the oil in a thin stream and process until the mayonnaise is thick and creamy. Season with salt and pepper and store as above.

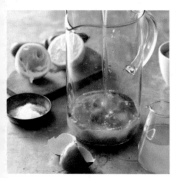 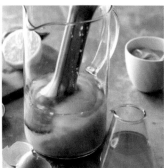 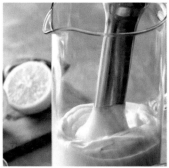 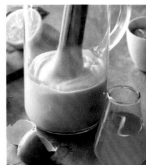

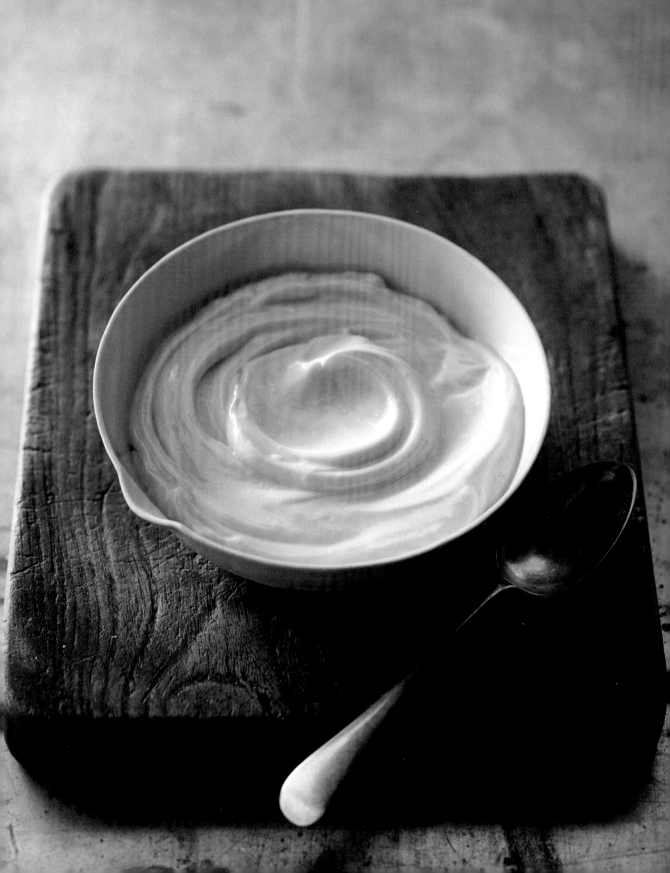

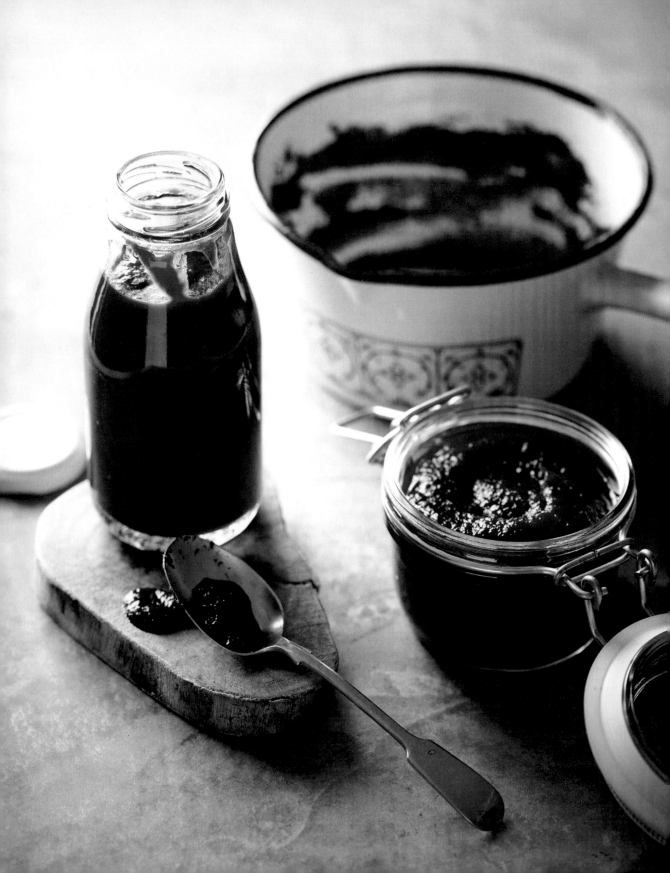

NOMATO SAUCE

Heat the fat in a large saucepan over medium heat. Add the onion and cook, stirring occasionally, until translucent. Add the garlic, carrots, and beets and cook for another 5 minutes, stirring occasionally.

Add the broth or filtered water, using only enough to cover the vegetables (you can add a little more after cooking and blending to reach the consistency you desire).

Add the dried herbs, bay leaf, and lemon juice and stir well to combine. Bring to a boil and simmer for about 30 to 40 minutes, until all the vegetables are very tender.

Remove the bay leaf and cool the mixture slightly before blending. Working in batches, carefully blend to a smooth puree. Add a little more liquid if needed to reach the desired consistency, and season with salt and pepper to taste. Store in the refrigerator for up to 5 days, or freeze for up to 3 months.

This sauce is great for any recipe that calls for Italian tomato sauce such as Bolognese or marinara. It's also delicious on top of parsnip spaghetti.

Makes: 2½ quarts

1 Tbsp duck fat, tallow, coconut oil, or other good-quality fat

½ large onion, chopped

2 cloves garlic, minced

6 large carrots, peeled and chopped

2 large beets, peeled and chopped

4 cups Chicken or Beef Bone Broth (see recipes, pages 77 and 87) or filtered water

2 tsp dried Italian herb mix

1 bay leaf

2 Tbsp lemon juice

Sea salt and freshly ground black pepper

SAUTEED BROCCOLI WITH SPICY MAYONNAISE

In this recipe, we are stepping up the vegetables and letting them take center stage. The key to this lifestyle is to keep it simple and fill your plate with low-carb vegetables, then add good fats and protein in the form of seafood, meat, or eggs. With this recipe, you have the vegetables and the fat component, so you just need to cook up a piece of fish or meat to serve alongside it. If you don't have time to make a sriracha sauce, simply add chili flakes, wasabi, horseradish, or your choice of herb to the mayo.

Serves: 4

2 heads broccoli, broken into florets

2 Tbsp coconut oil or good-quality animal fat

4 garlic cloves, chopped

2 long red chilies, seeded and thinly sliced

Sea salt and freshly ground black pepper

1 Tbsp extra-virgin olive oil

Lemon juice or apple cider vinegar, to serve (optional)

SPICY MAYONNAISE

1 Tbsp Sriracha Chili Sauce (see recipe opposite)

½ cup Mayonnaise (see recipe, page 236)

TO MAKE THE SPICY MAYONNAISE, place the sriracha chili sauce and mayonnaise in a bowl and mix to combine.

Blanch the broccoli in boiling salted water until tender, about 3 minutes, then immediately plunge into ice-cold water to stop the cooking process. When the broccoli is completely cold, drain well and set aside.

Heat the coconut oil in a wok or large frying pan over medium-high heat. Add the garlic and chilies, swirl around in the pan, and cook for 30 seconds, until fragrant. Add the broccoli and sauté, tossing occasionally, for 5 minutes, until it starts to color. Season with salt and pepper and drizzle over the olive oil.

If you like, squeeze a little lemon juice or pour a splash of vinegar over the sautéed broccoli for an extra boost of flavor. Serve with the spicy mayonnaise on the side or drizzled over the broccoli.

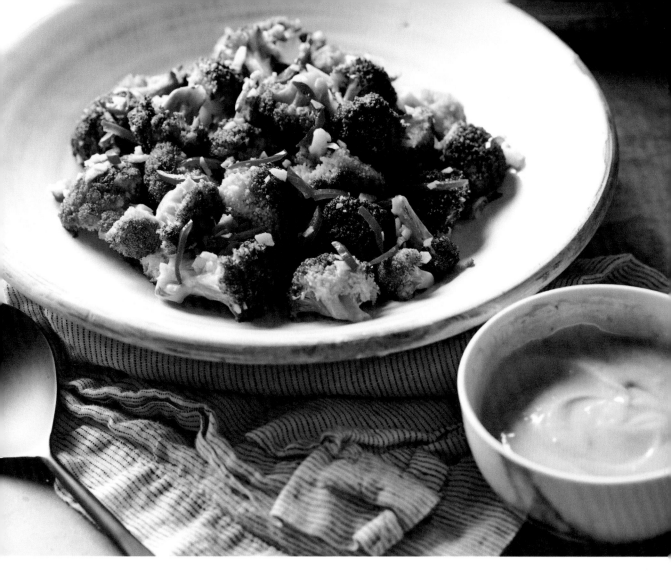

Combine all the ingredients in the bowl of a food processor and process until smooth. Pour into a saucepan and bring to a boil over high heat, stirring occasionally. Reduce the heat to low and simmer, stirring now and then, for 5 to 10 minutes, until the sauce is a vibrant red. Remove from the heat and cool. Transfer to a large, airtight glass jar and refrigerate for up to 2 weeks.

SRIRACHA CHILI SAUCE

Makes: 2 cups

1½ lb long red chilies, seeded and roughly chopped

8 garlic cloves, crushed

4 Tbsp apple cider vinegar

3 Tbsp tomato paste

1 large medjool date, pitted

2 Tbsp fish sauce

½ teaspoon sea salt

SHAVED ASPARAGUS SALAD WITH GREEN GODDESS DRESSING

If you are looking for a way to wow your guests, then look no further. Team this salad with grilled fish for a truly memorable dinner.

Serves: 4 as a side dish

¾ lb asparagus, woody ends trimmed

½ lb heirloom cherry tomatoes, cut into quarters

1 Lebanese cucumber, peeled, seeded, and finely diced

HERB DRESSING

1 Tbsp finely snipped chives

1 Tbsp finely chopped flat-leaf parsley

3 Tbsp lemon juice or apple cider vinegar

4 Tbsp extra-virgin olive oil

Sea salt and freshly ground black pepper

TO SERVE:

4 Tbsp Green Goddess Dressing (see recipe opposite)

3½ oz Macadamia Cheese (see recipe opposite)

Baby basil leaves

Using a vegetable peeler or mandoline, shave the asparagus into thin ribbons starting from the bottom end. Place the asparagus ribbons in one bowl and the tomatoes and cucumber in another bowl.

TO MAKE THE HERB DRESSING, combine the chives, parsley, lemon juice, and olive oil in a bowl and whisk well. Season with salt and pepper.

Pour half of the dressing over the asparagus and almost all of the remainder over the tomato and cucumber. Gently toss until evenly coated.

Arrange the asparagus on 4 serving plates, then top with the tomato and cucumber. Smear a tablespoon of green goddess dressing on each plate, then sprinkle with the macadamia cheese. Drizzle with the remainder of the herb dressing and finish with some basil leaves on top.

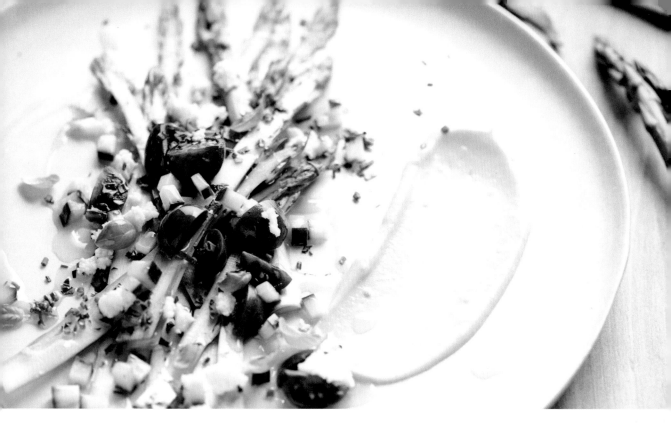

FOR THE GREEN GODDESS DRESSING, place all the ingredients except the oil in a food processor bowl and process until well combined. With the motor running, slowly pour in the oil and process until the dressing thickens and the herbs are finely chopped. Store in a glass jar in the fridge for up to 5 days.

TO MAKE THE MACADAMIA CHEESE, soak the macadamia nuts in 3¼ cups water for 6 hours. Drain and rinse well.

Place the nuts in a food processor with the lemon juice, salt, and pepper and pulse for 1 minute to combine. Add ½ cup of water and process until smooth. If the mixture seems a little dry, add more water and lemon juice to adjust the consistency. The macadamia cheese can be stored in an airtight container in the fridge for up to 1 week.

Makes: About 1⅓ cups

GREEN GODDESS DRESSING

Makes: About 1 cup

½ avocado, pitted and peeled

3 Tbsp coconut milk

3 Tbsp lemon juice

1 garlic clove, finely chopped

2 anchovy fillets, finely chopped

½ cup chopped flat-leaf parsley leaves

3 Tbsp chopped basil leaves

1 Tbsp chopped tarragon leaves

¼ tsp salt

½ cup extra-virgin olive oil

MACADAMIA CHEESE

1¼ cups macadamia nuts

1 to 1½ Tbsp lemon juice

1 tsp sea salt

Pinch freshly ground black pepper

SIMPLE BRAISED VEGETABLES

We all sometimes face the dilemma of what to do with leftover vegetables in the bottom of the fridge. Well, you need never worry again, as you can simply braise them until tender in a little bone broth. They are the perfect accompaniment to a roast. And for a delicious lunch, simply chill them and add some mayo, fresh herbs, animal protein (such as chicken, tuna, or salmon), and fermented vegetables.

Serves: 4

2 Tbsp coconut oil or good-quality animal fat

1 onion, cut into ½-inch wedges

3 garlic cloves, finely sliced

10 Dutch carrots, peeled and leafy ends trimmed

6 radishes, halved

3 turnips, cut into 1-inch pieces

¼ savoy cabbage, roughly chopped

1 green apple, cored and cut into 1-inch pieces

1 cup Chicken Bone Broth (see recipe, page 87) or water

2 bay leaves

Sea salt and freshly ground black pepper

Preheat the oven to 350°F.

Melt the oil in a large, flameproof casserole dish over medium heat. Add the onion and garlic and cook for 2 minutes until they start to color slightly.

Add the carrots, radishes, turnips, cabbage, and apple and cook, stirring occasionally, for 6 minutes, until they just start to color.

Pour in the broth, add the bay leaves, and season with salt and pepper. Cover with a lid or some foil and braise in the oven for 30 minutes, until the vegetables are tender. Transfer the braised vegetables to a platter and serve.

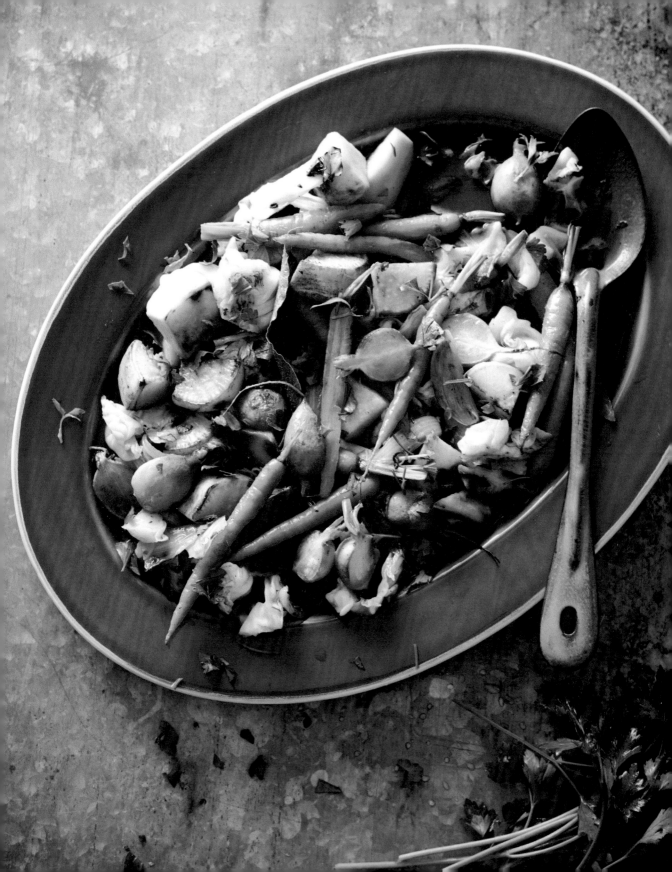

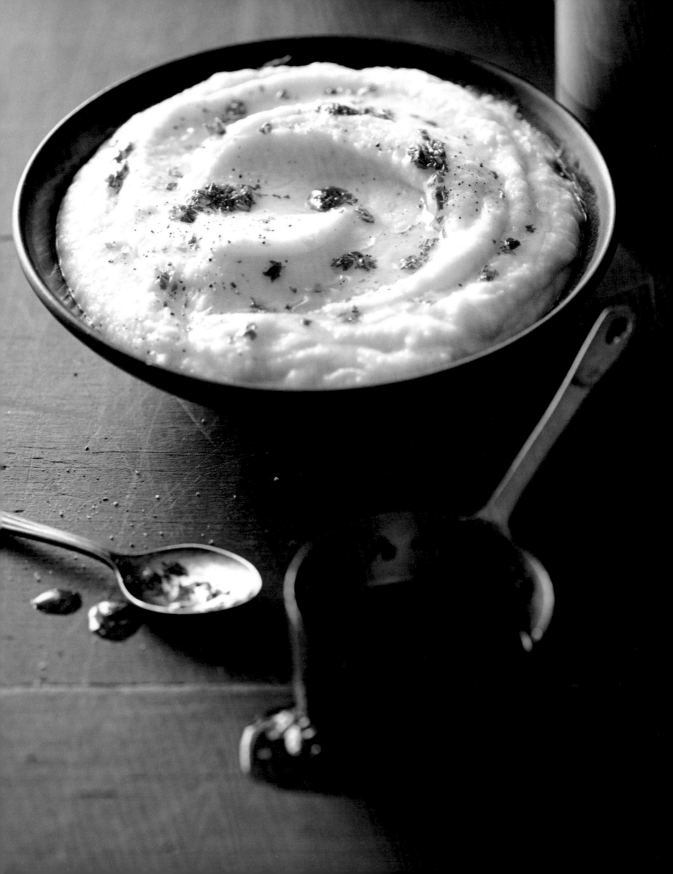

STEAMED CAULIFLOWER PUREE

This lovely creamy puree will become a regular part of your cooking repertoire after you have tried it. It's fantastic as a replacement for the old mashed potato, and the even greater news is that it is much quicker to cook, it won't elevate your blood sugar levels, and it works with everything from grilled seafood and meat to roasts, sausages, shepherd's and cottage pies, curries, and duck confit.

TO MAKE THE HERB OIL, combine the parsley, dill, and oil in a small bowl and mix well. Season with salt and pepper and set aside until needed.

Fill a saucepan with water and place a steamer with a lid on top. Bring to a boil, place the cauliflower florets in the steamer, cover, and steam for 30 to 35 minutes, until the cauliflower is very soft. Place the cauliflower in the bowl of a food processor and process until smooth. Add the oil or fat and blitz again, then season with salt and pepper.

Transfer the cauliflower puree to a serving bowl or plates and drizzle some herb oil over the top.

Serves: 4

1 large head organic cauliflower, chopped into florets

2 Tbsp coconut oil or good-quality animal fat, melted

HERB OIL

1 Tbsp finely chopped flat-leaf parsley

1 Tbsp finely chopped dill

3 Tbsp lemon-infused olive oil or extra-virgin olive oil

Sea salt and freshly ground black pepper

WHOLE ROASTED CABBAGE WITH BACON AND ONION BROTH

We all need to embrace getting more vegetables into our diet, and oven-roasting a whole cabbage is a ridiculously easy and fabulous way to celebrate the integrity and flavor of this humble vegetable while saving you a heap of time in the kitchen. For the perfect meal, try serving this with roast pork, pork cutlets, or some sausages. Any leftovers can be chopped or blended into chicken bone broth for the most amazing cabbage soup.

Serves: 6 to 8

4 Tbsp lard or other good-quality animal fat

2½ large onions, chopped

5 rindless bacon rashers, chopped

6 garlic cloves, chopped

1 tsp sweet paprika

2 Tbsp thyme leaves, chopped

½ cup white wine (such as chardonnay)

1 cabbage, outer dark green leaves removed

Sea salt and freshly ground black pepper

3 cups Chicken Bone Broth (see recipe, page 87)

3 Tbsp apple cider vinegar

1 small handful flat-leaf parsley, chopped

Preheat the oven to 325°F.

Place a large frying pan over medium heat. Add 3 tablespoons of the lard, then add the onions and sauté, stirring occasionally, for 8 minutes, until softened. Add the bacon and cook for 5 to 6 minutes, until the onions start to caramelize. Add the garlic, paprika, and thyme and sauté for 30 seconds, until fragrant. Add the wine, stir well, and cook until the liquid is almost completely gone. Set aside.

Place the cabbage in a large casserole dish. Rub the remaining 1 tablespoon lard over the cabbage and season well with salt and pepper. Add the broth and vinegar, then spoon over the bacon-and-onion mixture. Cover tightly with a lid or parchment paper and roast for 3½ hours, until the cabbage is cooked through. Increase the oven temperature to 350°F. Remove the lid or paper, baste the cabbage with some of the broth in the casserole dish, and return to the oven to roast for 30 minutes more, until golden. Sprinkle the parsley over the top and serve.

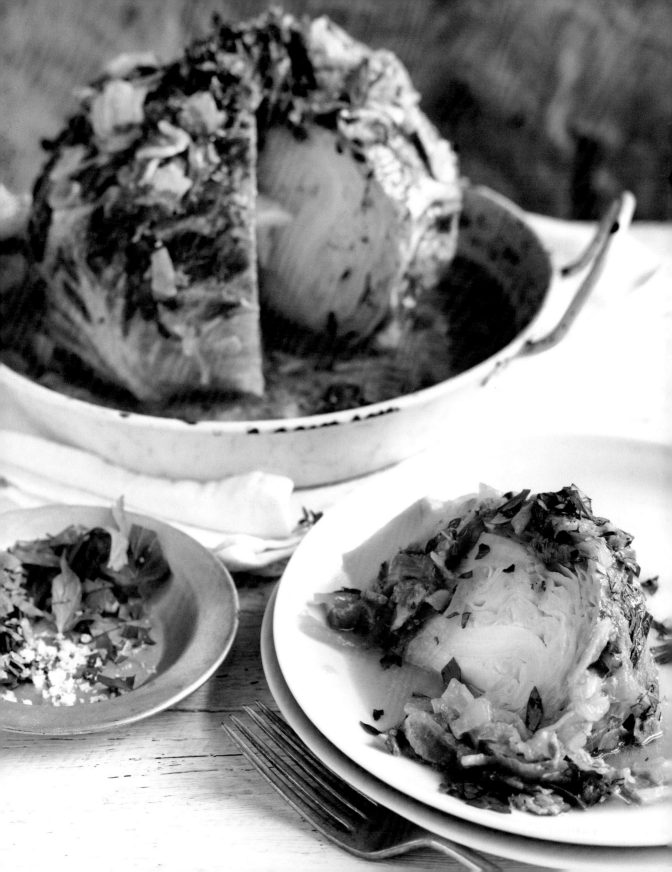

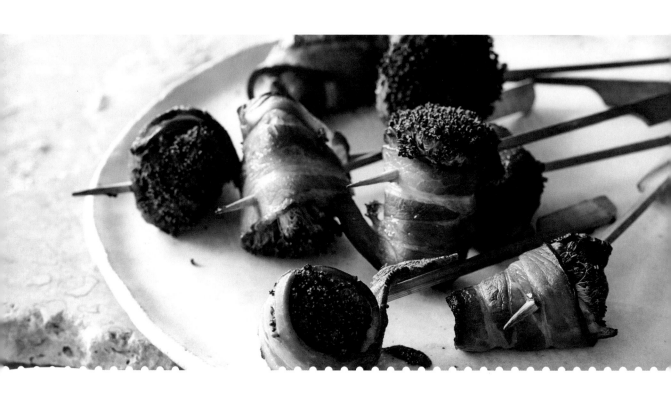

SNACKS AND TREATS

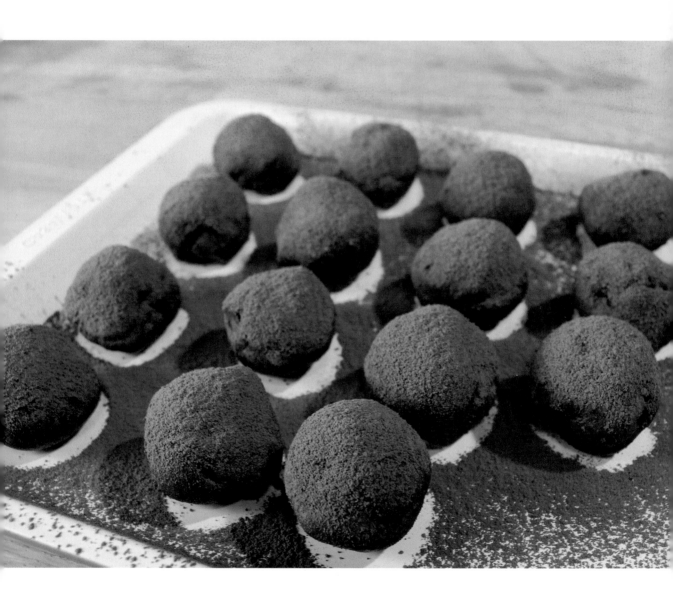

AVOCADO CHOCOLATE TRUFFLES

Chocolate truffles are a popular type of confectionery composed of a chocolate coating and ganache, a filling made by mixing chocolate and cream. The ingredients are mixed together and rolled into balls, which are then served as gifts or eaten for a quick snack.

However, most chocolate truffles sold today contain lots of sugar, which can wreak havoc on your health when consumed. I believe it's far better to make your own chocolate truffles using raw, organic ingredients that can provide a multitude of health benefits. Plus, it'll taste better, too!

This chocolate and avocado truffle recipe is based on a recipe by Jennafer Ashley of Paleohacks and is a great example. Not only is it healthy and delicious, but also easy to prepare.

In a mixing bowl, combine the melted coconut oil, avocados, honey, vanilla extract, and stevia (if using). Use a hand mixer on medium speed to mix the ingredients until smooth.

Gradually mix in the 1 cup of raw cacao powder until it completely combines with the other ingredients. Place in the freezer for 10 minutes.

Using a tablespoon, scoop out the mixture and roll it into balls. Dust with the remaining 2 tablespoons cacao powder. Chill in the refrigerator before serving.

Makes: 12 truffles

3 Tbsp Dr. Mercola's coconut oil, melted

2 small ripe organic avocados

1 Tbsp Dr. Mercola's raw honey or 1 Tbsp monk fruit sweetener

1 Tbsp Dr. Mercola's vanilla extract

1 to 2 drops of stevia (optional)

1 cup raw cacao powder plus 2 Tbsp for dusting

BROCCOLI SKEWERS

You can try this simple and tasty recipe with different types of vegetables. Cauliflower, mushrooms, asparagus, pumpkin, and Jerusalem artichokes all work well, but my all-time favorite has to be broccoli. You will need to soak 20 bamboo skewers in water for 10 minutes for this recipe.

Serves: 4 to 6

5 rindless streaky (from pork belly) bacon rashers, cut in half crossways, then halved lengthwise (optional)

1 head of broccoli, cut into 20 florets

1 Tbsp coconut oil or good-quality animal fat, melted

Sea salt and freshly ground black pepper

Juice of ½ lemon

½ cup Aioli (see recipe below)

2 pinches smoked paprika

AIOLI

6 garlic confit cloves (to make your own, see below)

4 egg yolks

2 tsp Dijon mustard

2 tsp apple cider vinegar

2 Tbsp lemon juice

1½ cups olive oil

Sea salt and freshly ground black pepper

GARLIC CONFIT

25 garlic cloves, peeled

1 cup coconut oil

Preheat the oven to 400°F. Line a baking tray with parchment paper.

If desired, wrap a bacon strip around each broccoli floret, then carefully insert a skewer through the bacon and broccoli to hold them together.

Place the skewers on the prepared tray in a single layer, approximately ½ inch apart to help them cook evenly. Drizzle with the oil and sprinkle on some salt and pepper. Bake for 20 minutes, until the broccoli is cooked through and the bacon is golden and crispy.

Transfer the skewers to a platter and squeeze some lemon juice over them. Spoon the aioli into a small serving bowl, sprinkle on the smoked paprika, and serve with the skewers.

TO MAKE YOUR OWN AIOLI, place the garlic cloves, egg yolks, mustard, vinegar, lemon juice, and some salt in a food processor and process until combined. With the motor running, slowly pour in the oil in a thin stream and process until the aioli is thick and creamy. Season with salt and pepper. Leftover aioli can be stored in an airtight container in the fridge for 4 to 5 days.

TO MAKE THE GARLIC CONFIT, place the garlic cloves and coconut oil in a small saucepan over very low heat (you do not want the oil to boil). Cook for 2 hours, or until the garlic is beautifully soft. Leftover garlic confit can be transferred to a sealed jar with the oil and stored in the fridge for up to 3 months.

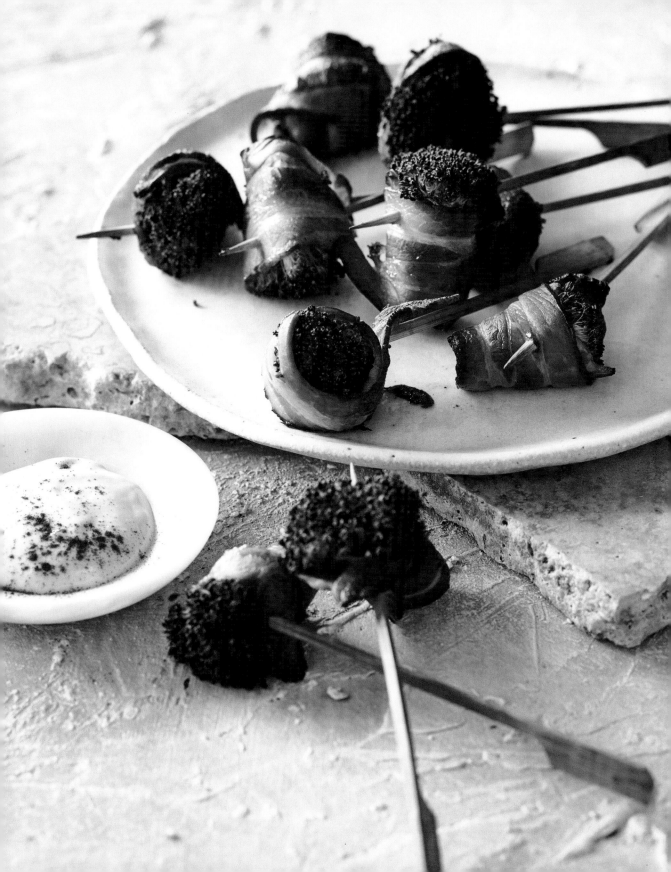

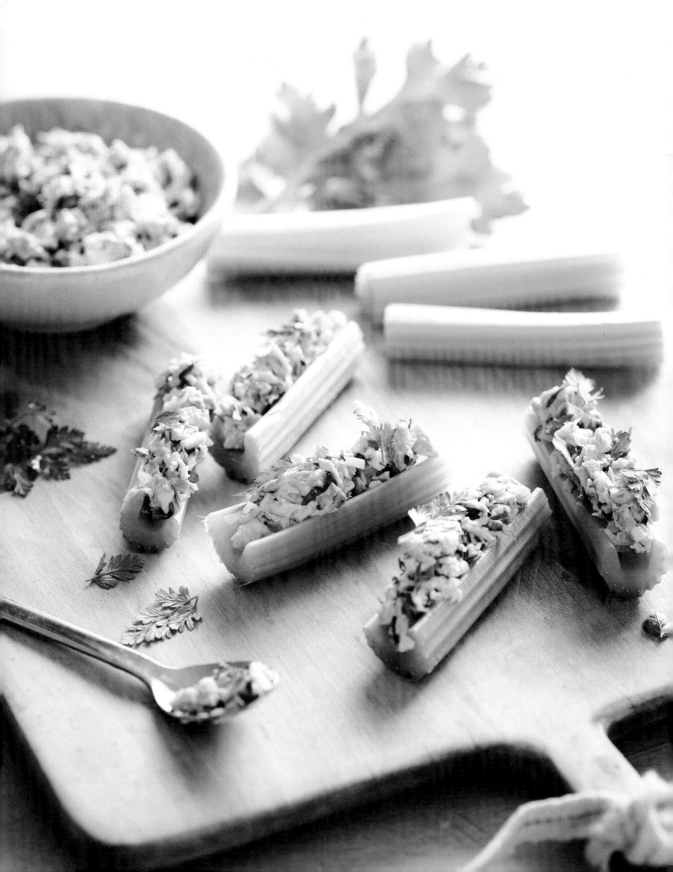

CHICKEN SALAD CELERY BOATS

Chefs use celery in so many preparations, as it is part of the classic mirepoix: a mix of onion, carrot, and celery that forms the basis of most French stocks and sauces. Celery is also sensational raw, in terms of both flavor and texture. Topping this beautiful vegetable with a simple chicken salad that has been mixed with creamy homemade mayonnaise is surely one of life's little luxuries. And the kids will love it too!

Using a vegetable peeler, peel the rounded undersides of the celery stalks so they sit flat, then cut them into 1½-inch pieces.

Place the remaining ingredients in a bowl and mix until combined. Season with salt and pepper to taste and add a little more lemon juice if desired.

To serve, spoon 1½ teaspoons of the chicken salad (add more if needed) onto each celery piece and garnish with chervil leaves.

Serves: 4

4 wide celery stalks, trimmed top and bottom

2 organic chicken thighs, cooked and finely chopped

4 Tbsp Mayonnaise (see recipe, page 236)

1 Tbsp lemon juice, plus extra if desired

1 tsp tarragon

1 Tbsp finely chopped flat-leaf parsley

½ tsp finely grated lemon zest

2 Tbsp finely chopped red onion

Sea salt and freshly ground black pepper

Chervil leaves, to serve

CHOCOLATE FAT BOMB

Apart from its delicious taste, this Chocolate Fat Bomb gives you moderate protein, low net carbs, and a healthy dose of fats. I don't consume this entire recipe in one sitting, though. I usually split it in half, so if you're eating this for the first time, try it this way.

Serves: 1 to 2

1 Tbsp organic black sesame seeds, soaked

1 Tbsp flax seeds

1 Tbsp organic black cumin seeds

1 Tbsp organic psyllium

1 Tbsp chia seeds, soaked, plus more to serve

2 scoops (6 grams) Mercola Organic Greens supplement

1 tsp calcium from ground-pastured eggshells

1 oz raw organic cocoa butter

1 whole avocado, pitted and peeled

1 Tbsp medium-chain triglyceride (MCT) oil

1 to 4 dropperfuls stevia (to desired sweetness)

1 to 2 oz fresh or frozen berries (optional)

Filtered water

Let the black sesame, flax, and black cumin seeds soak overnight (roughly 14 hours) in a mixing bowl or a 1-quart blender.

Add all remaining ingredients except the filtered water to the soaked seeds. Add some filtered water, then use an immersion blender (or Nutrabullet) to blend until the mixture reaches the desired consistency, adding more water if necessary. Consistency can range from a liquid to a pudding texture, depending on how much water you add.

Place in a serving bowl and sprinkle with extra chia seeds.

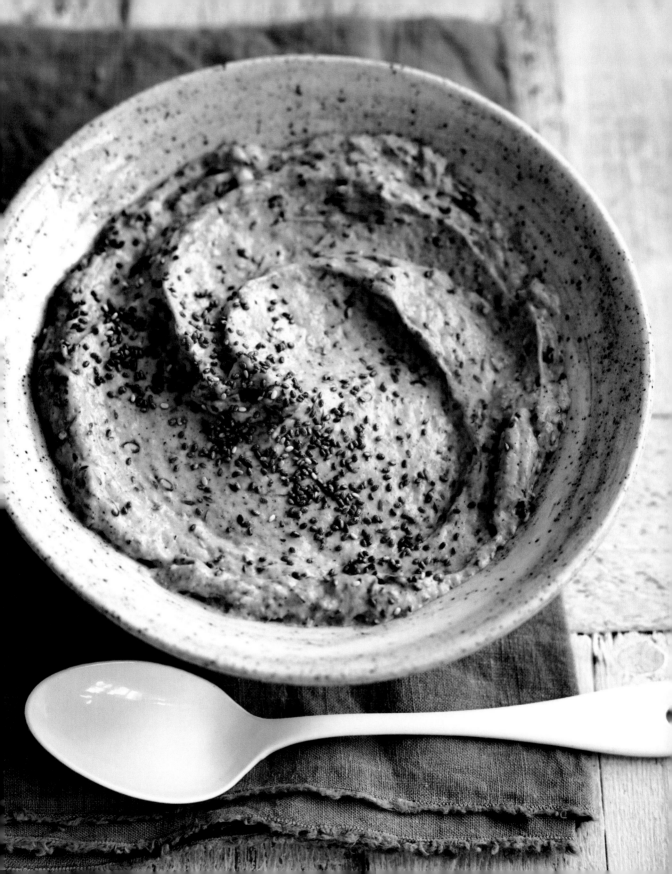

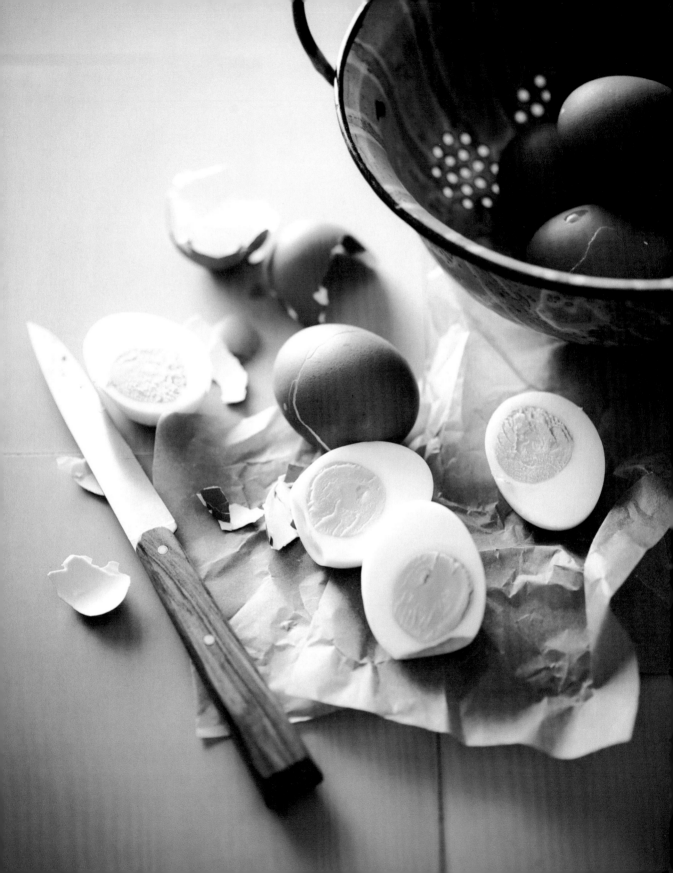

HARD-BOILED EGGS

Rich in protein and good fats, an egg or two will fill you up and stop you from snacking on unhealthier options. Boil up a dozen or so eggs at a time, depending on how many people there are in your family. Keep them in the fridge to snack on or to chop up and add to salads (they will last in the fridge for 7 days unpeeled or 5 days peeled).

If you want to get fancy, you can shave some truffle over your eggs, team them with caviar, or roll them in finely chopped activated nuts and seeds. For Pete, all it takes is salt, pepper, dried chili flakes, and some chopped herbs, and he is a happy man.

Bring a small saucepan of water to a boil over high heat.

Reduce the heat to low so that the water is simmering, then add the eggs and cook for 7 minutes. Drain. When cool enough to handle, peel the eggs under cold running water. Cut each egg in half and serve.

Serves: 2

4 organic, pasture-raised eggs (preferably from a local farmer)

KETO CHOCOLATE AND COCONUT BITES

What more is there to say than *yummy* when it comes to these tasty little morsels?

Makes: 15 to 20 pieces

3 Tbsp raw cacao powder, sifted

1 Tbsp carob powder

⅔ cup cacao butter, chopped

2 Tbsp coconut oil

¼ tsp vanilla extract

½ tsp liquid stevia (more if desired)

3 Tbsp coconut milk

Small pinch sea salt

3½ oz coconut flakes

Grease a mini muffin pan or chocolate mold tray.

Combine the cacao powder, carob powder, cacao butter, coconut oil, vanilla, and stevia in a heatproof bowl and place over a saucepan of simmering water. Make sure the bowl doesn't touch the water (or it will overheat). Stir with a metal spoon until smooth and the butters are just melted. Remove from the heat and stir in the coconut milk. Allow to cool to lukewarm, then stir in the salt and coconut flakes. Spoon the mixture evenly into the prepared muffin pan and place in the refrigerator for 1 hour, until firm.

Remove the pan from the fridge, tap the base of the pan on your countertop a couple of times, then flip over to remove the bites. They should pop out easily, but if they don't, try tapping the pan again on the countertop. Store in an airtight container in the fridge.

TIP: You can add a couple of drops of food-grade essential oils, such as orange or spearmint, to these bites. Food-grade essential oils can be purchased from health food stores or online.

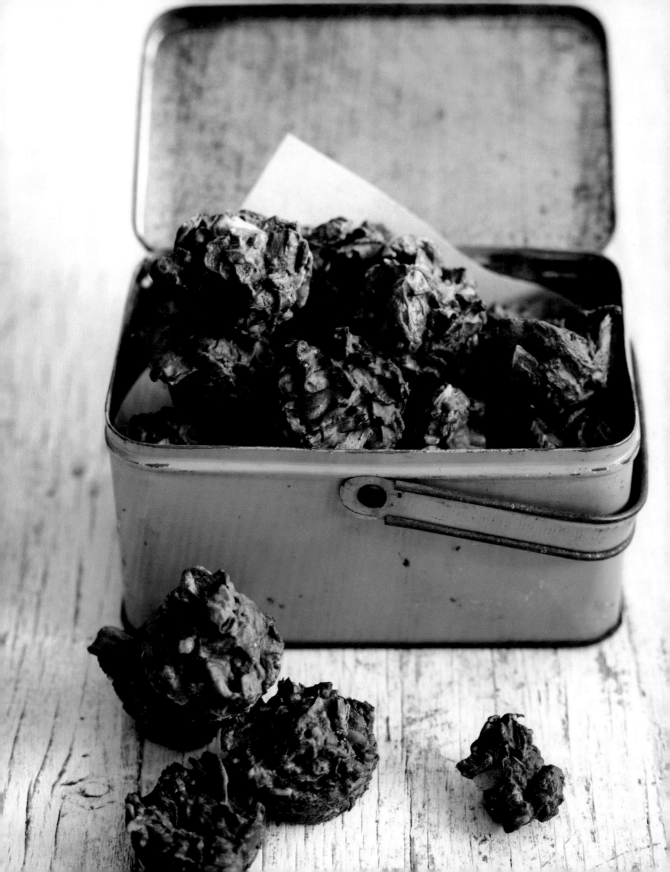

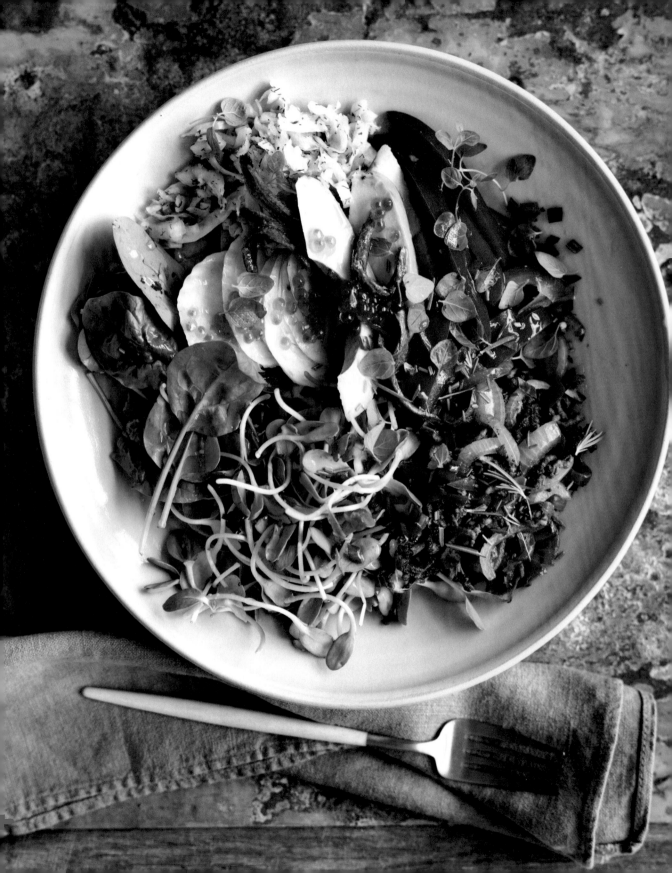

KETO SALAD

As you know, I enjoy making my own meals, experimenting with different ingredients, most of which are from my garden. One of my favorite lunch recipes is my signature keto salad, a meal with high amounts of beneficial fat, moderate amounts of high-quality protein, and no starchy vegetable carbohydrates.

Gently heat the coconut oil in a small frying pan over low heat. Add onion and meat, if not using sardines, and cook, stirring occasionally, until onion and meat are cooked as desired. Season with salt and pepper.

Meanwhile, in a separate medium bowl, combine the avocado, salmon roe, fennel, spinach, herbs, sprouts, and fermented vegetables.

Rinse the sardines and soak them for five minutes in cold filtered water. Drain and cut each sardine into three pieces and add to the salad.

Add the cooked onion and meat, if using, to the salad.

Mix gently and season with salt and pepper.

Serves: 2

1 to 2 Tbsp extra-virgin coconut oil or raw organic pastured butter

⅓ medium red onion, chopped

One 3.75-oz can sardines in water, or 2.5 oz cleaned shrimp, or 2.5 oz organic, pastured ground meat

1 avocado, pitted, peeled, and sliced

1 Tbsp salmon roe

1 oz chopped fresh fennel, or more if desired

Handful spinach (preferably Malabar when in season)

2 sprigs fresh rosemary, leaves chopped finely

Handful fresh oregano leaves

2 to 4 oz sunflower seed sprouts

3 oz fermented vegetables of your choice

Himalayan salt and freshly ground black pepper

MACADAMIA NUT FUDGE

Many of you have also asked what I regularly eat, so I'd like to share with you one of my favorite healthy treats, my very own Macadamia Nut Fudge. It's one of the recipes featured in my "A Day in the Life" video on Mercola.com.

This snack is made of all-natural ingredients and is loaded with healthy fats and nutrients that make it a great complement to the other foods I eat throughout the day.

Serves: 8

10½ oz cocoa butter, chopped

1 cup coconut oil

10½ oz raw, organic, pastured butter or ghee or coconut oil

4 to 8 dropperfuls stevia (or substitute monk fruit) to desired taste

1 tsp organic vanilla extract

2¼ cups whole macadamia nuts

Place the cocoa butter, coconut oil, and butter in a saucepan and gently melt over low heat. Remove from the heat and allow to cool to lukewarm.

Once the mixture has cooled, add the stevia and vanilla extract and stir to combine.

Pour the fudge into 8-oz wide-mouth Ball jars or a flan tin. Spread the nuts evenly across all jars or the flan tin. Refrigerate until the fudge reaches the desired consistency.

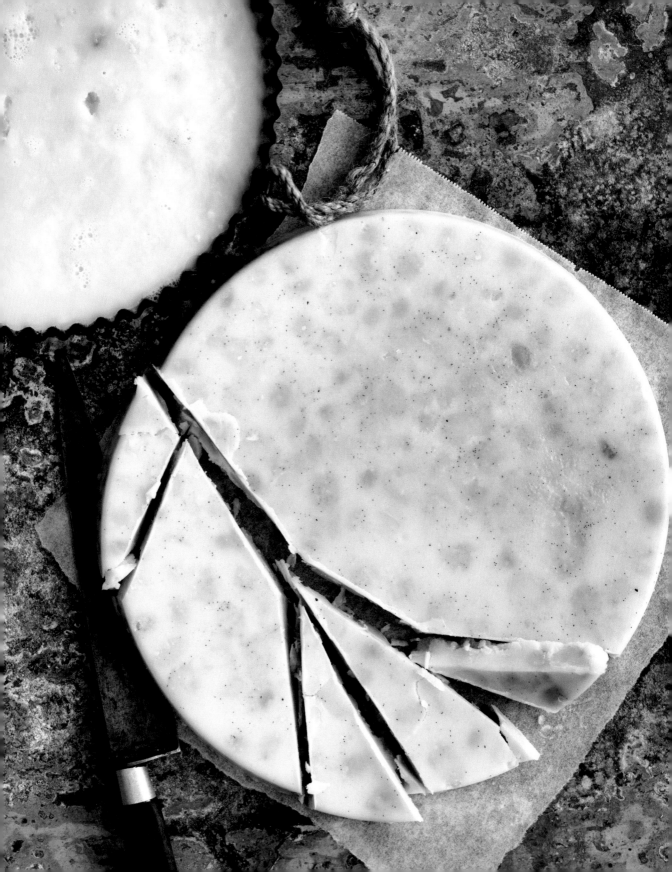

METRIC CONVERSION CHART

The recipes in this book use the standard United States method for measuring liquid and dry or solid ingredients (teaspoons, tablespoons, and cups). The following charts are provided to help cooks outside the U.S. successfully use these recipes. All equivalents are approximate.

Standard Cup	Fine Powder (e.g., flour)	Grain (e.g., rice)	Granular (e.g., sugar)	Liquid Solids (e.g., butter)	Liquid (e.g., milk)
1	140 g	150 g	190 g	200 g	240 ml
¾	105 g	113 g	143 g	150 g	180 ml
⅔	93 g	100 g	125 g	133 g	160 ml
½	70 g	75 g	95 g	100 g	120 ml
⅓	47 g	50 g	63 g	67 g	80 ml
¼	35 g	38 g	48 g	50 g	60 ml
⅛	18 g	19 g	24 g	25 g	30 ml

Useful Equivalents for Liquid Ingredients by Volume				
¼ tsp			1 ml	
½ tsp			2 ml	
1 tsp			5 ml	
3 tsp	1 tbsp		½ fl oz	15 ml
	2 tbsp	⅛ cup	1 fl oz	30 ml
	4 tbsp	¼ cup	2 fl oz	60 ml
	5⅓ tbsp	⅓ cup	3 fl oz	80 ml
	8 tbsp	½ cup	4 fl oz	120 ml
	10⅔ tbsp	⅔ cup	5 fl oz	160 ml
	12 tbsp	¾ cup	6 fl oz	180 ml
	16 tbsp	1 cup	8 fl oz	240 ml
	1 pt	2 cups	16 fl oz	480 ml
	1 qt	4 cups	32 fl oz	960 ml
			33 fl oz	1000 ml 1 L

Useful Equivalents for Dry Ingredients by Weight

(To convert ounces to grams, multiply the number of ounces by 30.)

1 oz	¹⁄₁₆ lb	30 g
4 oz	¼ lb	120 g
8 oz	½ lb	240 g
12 oz	¾ lb	360 g
16 oz	1 lb	480 g

Useful Equivalents for Cooking/Oven Temperatures

Process	Fahrenheit	Celsius	Gas Mark
Freeze Water	32° F	0° C	
Room Temperature	68° F	20° C	
Boil Water	212° F	100° C	
Bake	325° F	160° C	3
	350° F	180° C	4
	375° F	190° C	5
	400° F	200° C	6
	425° F	220° C	7
	450° F	230° C	8
Broil			Grill

Useful Equivalents for Length

(To convert inches to centimeters, multiply the number of inches by 2.5.)

1 in			2.5 cm	
6 in	½ ft		15 cm	
12 in	1 ft		30 cm	
36 in	3 ft	1 yd	90 cm	
40 in			100 cm	1 m

ENDNOTES

INTRODUCTION

1. K. M. Adams, W. S. Butsch, and M. Kohlmeier, "The State of Nutrition Education at US Medical Schools," *Journal of Biomedical Education* 2015 (January 2015), Article ID 357627. DOI:10.1155/2015/357627.

CHAPTER 1

1. W. S. Yancy, Jr., et al., "A Low-Carbohydrate, Ketogenic Diet versus a Low-Fat Diet to Treat Obesity and Hyperlipidemia: A Randomized, Controlled Trial," *Annals of Internal Medicine* 140, no. 10 (2004): 769–777. DOI: 10.7326/0003-4819-140-10-200405180-00006.

2. F. J. McClernon, et al., "The Effects of a Low-Carbohydrate Ketogenic Diet and a Low-Fat Diet on Mood, Hunger, and Other Self-Reported Symptoms," *Obesity* 15, no. 1 (2007): 182–187.

3. E. C. Westman, et al., "The Effect of a Low-Carbohydrate, Ketogenic Diet versus a Low-Glycemic Index Diet on Glycemic Control in Type 2 Diabetes Mellitus," *Nutrition & Metabolism* 5, no. 36 (2008): 36. DOI: 10.1186/1743-7075-5-36.

CHAPTER 2

1. R. Sender, S. Fuchs, and R. Milo, "Revised Estimates for the Number of Human and Bacterial Cells in the Body," *PLoS Biology* 14, no. 8 (2016): e1002533. DOI:10.1371/journal.pbio.1002533.

2. L. M. Cox, et al., "Altering the Intestinal Microbiota during a Critical Developmental Window Has Lasting Metabolic Consequences," *Cell* 158, no. 4 (2014): 705–721. DOI: 10.1016/j.cell.2014.05.052.

3. C. Potera, "POPs and Gut Microbiota: Dietary Exposure Alters Ratio of Bacterial Species," *Environmental Health Perspectives* 123, no. 7 (2015). DOI: 10.1289/ehp.123-A187.

4. M. C. Dao, J. Everard, J. Aron-Wisnewsky, et al., "*Akkermansia muciniphila* and Improved Metabolic Health during a Dietary Intervention in Obesity: Relationship with Gut Microbiome Richness and Ecology," *Gut* 65, no. 3 (2016): 426–436. DOI: 10.1136/gutjnl-2014-308778.

5. P. Hemarajata and J. Versalovic, "Effects of Probiotics on Gut Microbiota: Mechanisms of Intestinal Immunomodulation and Neuromodulation," *Therapeutic Advances in Gastroenterology* 6, no. 1 (2013): 39–51.

6. K. R. Magnusson, et al., "Relationships between Diet-Related Changes in the Gut Microbiome and Cognitive Flexibility," *Neuroscience* 300 (2015): 128–140. DOI: 10.1016/j.neuroscience.2015.05.016.

7. M. R. Hillmire, et al., "Fermented Foods, Neuroticism, and Social Anxiety: An Interaction Model," *Psychiatry Research* 228, no. 2 (2015): 203–208. DOI: 10.1016/j.psychres.2015.04.023.

8. J. A. Bravo, et al., "Ingestion of *Lactobacillus* Strain Regulates Emotional Behavior and Central GABA Receptor Expression in a Mouse via the Vagus Nerve," *Proceedings of the National Academy of Sciences of the United States of America* 108, no. 38 (2011): 16050–16055. DOI: 10.1073/pnas.1102999108.

9. L. Steenbergen and R. Sellaro, "A Randomized Controlled Trial to Test the Effect of Multispecies Probiotics on Cognitive Reactivity to Sad Mood," *Brain, Behavior, and Immunity* 48 (2015): 258–264. DOI: 10.1016/j.bbi.2015.04.003.

10. BBC News, "Scientists Sniffing Out the Western Allergy Epidemic," August 27, 2014, http://www.bbc.com/news/health-28934415#, accessed 5/19/16.

11. S. W. Kembel, et al., "Architectural Design Influences the Diversity and Structure of the Built Environment Microbiome," *The ISME Journal* 6, no. 8 (2012): 1469–1479. DOI: 10.1038/ismej.2011.211.

CHAPTER 3

1. Centers for Disease Control and Prevention, "National Diabetes Statistics Report: Estimates of Diabetes and Its Burden in the United States, 2014," https://stacks.cdc.gov/view/cdc/23442, accessed 12/2/16.

2. Y. Huang, X. Cai, M. Qiu, et al., "Prediabetes and the Risk of Cancer: A Meta-Analysis," *Diabetologia* 57, no. 11 (2014): 2261–2269. DOI: 10.1007/s00125-014-3361-2.

3. J. W. Anderson, et al., "Health Benefits of Dietary Fiber," *Nutrition Reviews* 67, no. 4 (2009): 188–205. DOI: 10.1111/j.1753-4887.2009.00189.x.

4. M. Herrmann, et al., "Serum 25-Hydroxy Vitamin D: A Predictor of Macrovascular and Microvascular Complications in Patients with Type 2 Diabetes," *Diabetes Care* 38, no. 3 (2015): 521–528. DOI: 10.2337/dc14-0180.

5. C. Gibbons, M. Dempster, and M. Moutray, "Stress, Coping, and Satisfaction in Nursing Students," *Journal of Advanced Nursing* 67, no. 3 (2011): 621–632. DOI: 10.1111/j.1365-2648.2010.05495.x.

6. D. S. Schade and R. P. Eaton, "The Temporal Relationship between Endogenously Secreted Stress Hormones and Metabolic Decompensation in Diabetic Man," *Journal of Clinical Endocrinology and Metabolism* 50, no. 1 (1980): 131.6.

7. D.-J. Dijk, "Slow-Wave Sleep, Diabetes, and the Sympathetic Nervous System," *Proceedings of the National Academy of Sciences of the United States of America* 105, no. 4 (2008): 1107–1108. DOI: 10.1073/pnas.0711635105.

8. M. Herrmann, et al., "Serum 25-Hydroxy Vitamin D."

9. C. Dalgard, et al., "Vitamin D Status in Relation to Glucose Metabolism and Type 2 Diabetes in Septuagenarians," *Diabetes Care* 34, no. 6 (2011): 1284–1288. DOI: 10.2337/dc10-2084.

10. J. Parker, et al., "Levels of Vitamin D and Cardiometabolic Disorders: Systematic Review and Meta-analysis," *Maturitas* 65, no. 3 (2010): 225–236. DOI: 10.1016/j.maturitas.2009.12.013.

CHAPTER 4

1. L. Yang and G. A. Colditz, "Prevalence of Overweight and Obesity in the United States, 2007–2012," *JAMA Internal Medicine* 175, no. 8 (2015): 1412–1413. DOI: 10.1001/jamainternmed.2015.2405.

2. F. A. Kummerow, "Two Lipids in the Diet, Rather Than Cholesterol, Are Responsible for Heart Failure and Stroke," *Clinical Lipidology* 9, no. 2 (2014): 189–204. DOI: 10.2217/clp.14.4.

3. K. Kavanagh, et al., "Trans Fat Diet Induces Abdominal Obesity and Changes in Insulin Sensitivity in Monkeys," *Obesity* 15 (2007): 1675–1684. DOI: 10.1038/oby.2007.200.

4. Office of Disease Prevention and Health Promotion, "Dietary Guidelines," https://health.gov/dietaryguidelines/, accessed 5/25/17.

5. L. A. Tellez, et al. "Glucose Utilization Rates Regulate Intake Levels of Artificial Sweeteners," *The Journal of Physiology* 591, no. 22 (2013): 5727–5744. DOI: 10.1113/jphysiol.2013.263103.

6. J. Suez, et al., "Artificial Sweeteners Induce Glucose Intolerance by Altering the Gut Microbiota," *Nature* 514 (2014): 181–186. DOI: 10.1038/nature13793.

7. S. Fowler, K. Williams, and H. P. Hazuda, "Diet Soda Intake Is Associated with Long-Term Increases in Waist Circumference in a Biethnic Cohort of Older Adults: The San Antonio Longitudinal Study of Aging," *Journal of the American Geriatrics Society* 63, no. 4 (2015): 708–715. DOI: 10.1111/jgs.13376.

8. R. Jaslow, "New Study Is Wake-Up Call for Diet Soda Drinkers," CBS News, December 8, 2011, http://www.cbsnews.com/news/new-study-is-wake-up-call-for-diet-soda-drinkers/, accessed 8/9/17.

CHAPTER 5

1. Sugar Science: The Unsweetened Truth, "Hidden in Plain Sight," University of California San Francisco, http://sugarscience.ucsf.edu/hidden-in-plain-sight/#.WSwnBYVGqTM, accessed 5/29/17.

2. U.S. Department of Agriculture, "Sugar and Sweeteners Yearbook Tables, Table 51," https://www.ers.usda.gov/webdocs/DataFiles/53304/table51.xls?v=42538, accessed 5/29/17.

3. United States Department of Agriculture, "Sugar and Sweeteners Yearbook Tables, Table 52," https://www.ers.usda.gov/webdocs/DataFiles/53304/table52.xls?v=42538, accessed 5/29/17.

4. U.S. Department of Agriculture and U.S. Department of Health and Human Services, *Dietary Guidelines for Americans, 2010,* 7th Edition (Washington, DC: U.S. Government Printing Office, December 2010), https://health.gov/dietaryguidelines/dga2010/DietaryGuidelines2010.pdf, accessed 5/29/17.

5. K. L. Stanhope, et al., "Consuming Fructose-Sweetened, Not Glucose-Sweetened, Beverages Increases Visceral Adiposity and Lipids and Decreases Insulin Sensitivity in Overweight/Obese Humans," *The Journal of Clinical Investigation* 119, no. 5 (2009): 1322–1334. DOI: 10.1172/JCI37385.

6. The Cornucopia Institute, "Culture Wars: How the Food Giants Turned Yogurt, a Health Food, into Junk Food," November 2014, https://www.cornucopia.org/Yogurt-docs/CultureWars-FullReport.pdf, accessed 5/29/17.

7. U.S. Department of Agriculture, "Recent Trends in GE Adoption," https://www.ers.usda.gov/data-products/adoption-of-genetically-engineered-crops-in-the-us/recent-trends-in-ge-adoption.aspx, accessed 5/29/17.

8. L. E. Glynn, *Plant Lectins* (Cambridge: Cambridge University Press, 1992).

9. E. J. Brandt, et al., "Hospital Admissions for Myocardial Infarction and Stroke Before and After the Trans-Fatty Acid Restrictions in New York," *JAMA Cardiology*, published online April 12, 2017. DOI: 10.1001/jamacardio.2017.0491.

10. J. E. Brody, "The Worst Fat in the Food Supply," *The New York Times*, May 22, 2017.

11. J. Fernandez-Cornejo, et al., "Pesticide Use in U.S. Agriculture: 21 Selected Crops, 1960–2008," U.S. Department of Agriculture, Economic Information Bulletin no. 24, May 2014.

12. U.S. Food & Drug Administration, "You Can Help Cut Acrylamide in Your Diet," March 14, 2016, https://www.fda.gov/ForConsumers/ConsumerUpdates/ucm374855.htm, accessed 6/19/17.

13. M. Wien, et al., "A Randomized 3x3 Crossover Study to Evaluate the Effect of Hass Avocado Intake on Post-ingestive Satiety, Glucose and Insulin Levels, and Subsequent Energy Intake in Overweight Adults," *Nutrition Journal* 12 (2013): 155, DOI: 10.1186/1475-2891-12-155.

14. E. A. Lee, et al., "Targeting Mitochondria with Avocatin B Induces Selective Leukemia Cell Death," *Cancer Research* 75, no. 12 (June 15, 2015): 2478–2488. DOI: 10.1158/0008-5472.CAN-14-2676.

15. J. M. Lattimer and M. D. Haub, "Effects of Dietary Fiber and Its Components on Metabolic Health," *Nutrients* 2, no. 12 (2010): 1266–1289. DOI:10.3390/nu2121266.

16. G. Mithieux and A. Gautier-Stein, "Intestinal Glucose Metabolism Revisited," *Diabetes Research and Clinical Practice* 105, no. 3 (2014): 295–301. DOI: 10.1016/j.diabres.2014.04.008.

CHAPTER 6

1. J. Peretz, et al., "Bisphenol A and Reproductive Health: Update of Experimental and Human Evidence, 2007–2013," *Environmental Health Perspectives* 122, no. 8 (2014): 775–786. DOI: 10.1289/ehp.1307728.

2. E. L. Roen, et al., "Bisphenol A Exposure and Behavioral Problems among Inner City Children at 7–9 Years of Age," *Environmental Research* 142 (2015): 739–745.

3. J. Y. Youn, "Evaluation of the Immune Response Following Exposure of Mice to Bisphenol A: Induction of Th1 Cytokine and Prolactin by BPA Exposure in the Mouse Spleen Cells," *Archives of Pharmacal Research* 25, no. 6 (2002): 946–953.

4. G. S. Prins, et al., "Bisphenol A Promotes Human Prostate Stem-Progenitor Cell Self-Renewal and Increases In Vivo Carcinogenesis in Human Prostate Epithelium," *Endocrinology* 155, no. 3 (2014): 805–817. DOI: 10.1210/en.2013-1955.

5. M. Pupo, et al., "Bisphenol A Induces Gene Expression Changes and Proliferative Effects through GPER in Breast Cancer Cells and Cancer-Associated Fibroblasts," *Environmental Health Perspectives* 120, no. 8 (2012): 1177–1182. DOI: 10.1289/ehp.1104526.

6. P. Factor-Litvak, "Persistent Associations between Maternal Prenatal Exposure to Phthalates on Child IQ at Age 7 Years," *PLoS ONE* 9, no. 12 (2014): e114003. DOI: 10.1371/journal.pone.0114003.

7. A. Postman, "The Truth About Tap," Natural Resources Defense Council, January 5, 2016, https://www.nrdc.org/stories/truth-about-tap, accessed 5/29/17.

8. Y. Choi, Y. Chang, S. Ryu, et al, "Coffee Consumption and Coronary Artery Calcium in Young and Middle-Aged Asymptomatic Adults," *Heart* (2015). DOI:10.1136/heartjnl-2014-306663.

9. E. Loftfield, et al., "Coffee Drinking and Cutaneous Melanoma Risk in the NIH-AARP Diet and Health Study," *Journal of the National Cancer Institute* 107, no. 2 (2015): dju421. DOI: 10.1093/jnci/dju421.

10. F. Song, A. A. Qureshi, and J. Han, "Increased Caffeine Intake Is Associated with Reduced Risk of Basal Cell Carcinoma of the Skin," *Cancer Research* 72, no. 13 (2012). DOI: 10.1158/0008-5472.CAN-11-3511.

11. E. Mowry, et al., "Greater Consumption of Coffee Is Associated with Reduced Odds of Multiple Sclerosis," research presented at the American Academy of Neurology 67th Annual Meeting, February 2015, https://www.aan.com/PressRoom/Home/GetDigitalAsset/11535, accessed 5/29/17.

12. C. Cao, "High Blood Caffeine Levels in MCI Linked to Lack of Progression to Dementia," *Journal of Alzheimer's Disease* 30, no. 3 (2012): 559–572. DOI: 10.3233/JAD-2012-111781.

13. G. W. Ross, et al., "Association of Coffee and Caffeine Intake with the Risk of Parkinson Disease," *JAMA* 283, no. 20 (2000): 2674–2679. DOI: 10.1001/jama.283.20.2674.

14. C. Kotyczka, et al., "Dark Roast Coffee Is More Effective Than Light Roast Coffee in Reducing Body Weight, and in Restoring Red Blood Cell Vitamin E and Glutathione Concentrations in Healthy Volunteers," *Molecular Nutrition & Food Research* 55, no. 10 (2011): 1582–1586. DOI: 10.1002/mnfr.201100248.

CHAPTER 7

1. S. M. Ulven, et al., "Metabolic Effects of Krill Oil Are Essentially Similar to Those of Fish Oil but at Lower Dose of EPA and DHA, in Healthy Volunteers," *Lipids* 46, no. 1 (2011): 37–46. DOI: 10.1007/s11745 -010-3490-4.

2. D. Piovesan, et al., "The Human 'Magnesome': Detecting Magnesium Binding Sites on Human Proteins," *BMC Bioinformatics* 13, suppl. 14 (2012): S10. DOI: 10.1186/1471-2105-13-S14-S10.

3. University of Maryland Medical Center, "Zinc," https://umm.edu/health/medical/altmed/supplement/zinc, accessed 6/14/17.

4. J. Teas, et al., "Dietary Seaweed Modifies Estrogen and Phytoestrogen Metabolism in Healthy Postmenopausal Women," *Journal of Nutrition* 139, no. 5 (2009): 939–944. DOI: 10.3945/jn.108.100834.

5. Y. J. Yang, et al., "A Case-Control Study on Seaweed Consumption and the Risk of Breast Cancer," *British Journal of Nutrition* 103, no. 9 (2010): 1345–1353. DOI: 10.1017/S0007114509993242.

6. R. L. Bailey, et al., "Multivitamin-Mineral Use Is Associated with Reduced Risk of Cardiovascular Disease Mortality among Women in the United States," *Journal of Nutrition* 145, no. 3 (2015): 572–578. DOI: 10.3945/jn.114.204743.

CHAPTER 8

1. National Cancer Institute, "Chemicals in Meat Cooked at High Temperatures and Cancer Risk," https://www.cancer.gov/about-cancer/causes-prevention/risk/diet/cooked-meats-fact-sheet, accessed 6/21/17.

2. T. Sugimura, K. Wakabayashi, H. Nakagama, and M. Nagao, "Heterocyclic Amines: Mutagens/Carcinogens Produced during Cooking of Meat and Fish," *Cancer Science* 95 (2004): 290–299. DOI: 10.1111/j.1349-7006.2004.tb03205.x.

3. K. Puangsombat, et al., "Occurrence of Heterocyclic Amines in Cooked Meat Products," *Meat Science* 90, no. 3 (2012): 739–746. DOI: 10.1016/j.meatsci.2011.11.005.

4. J. Uribarri, et al., "Advanced Glycation End Products in Foods and a Practical Guide to Their Reduction in the Diet," *Journal of the American Dietetic Association* 110, no. 6 (2010): 911–916.e12. DOI: 10.1016/j.jada.2010.03.018.

5. O. Sandu, et al., "Insulin Resistance and Type 2 Diabetes in High-Fat–Fed Mice Are Linked to High Glycotoxin Intake," *Diabetes* 54, no. 8 (2005): 2314–2319. DOI: 10.2337/diabetes.54.8.2314.

6. F. Zheng, et al., "Prevention of Diabetic Nephropathy in Mice by a Diet Low in Glycoxidation Products," *Diabetes/Metabolism Research and Review* 18 (2002): 224–237. DOI: 10.1002/dmrr.283.

7. R.-Y. Lin, et al., "Dietary Glycotoxins Promote Diabetic Atherosclerosis in Apolipoprotein E-deficient Mice," *Atherosclerosis* 168, no. 2 (2003): 213–220. DOI: 10.1016/S0021-9150(03)00050-9.

8. M. Peppa, et al., "Adverse Effects of Dietary Glycotoxins on Wound Healing in Genetically Diabetic Mice," *Diabetes* 52, no. 11 (2003): 2805–2813. DOI: 10.2337/diabetes.52.11.2805.

9. J. Uribarri, et al., "Advanced Glycation End Products in Foods."

10. Ibid.

11. Committee on Diet, Nutrition, and Cancer, Assembly of Life Sciences, National Research Council, *Diet, Nutrition and Cancer* (Washington, D.C.: National Academy Press, 1982), http://www.nap.edu/openbook.php?record_id=371&page=1, accessed 9/27/10.

12. J. Schor, "Marinades Reduce Heterocyclic Amines from Primitive Food Preparation Techniques," *Natural Medicine Journal* 2, no. 7 (2010).

13. Ibid.

14. Ibid.

15. F. Vallejo, F. Tomás-Barberán, and C. García-Viguera, "Phenolic Compound Contents in Edible Parts of Broccoli Inflorescences after Domestic Cooking," *Journal of the Science of Food and Agriculture* 83 (2003): 1511–1516. DOI: 10.1002/jsfa.1585.

16. K. Song and J. A. Milner, "The Influence of Heating on the Anticancer Properties of Garlic," *Journal of Nutrition* 131, no. 3s (2001): 1054S–1057S.

17. J. Gornall, "Is It Safe to Microwave Food in Plastic?" *The Daily Mail*, November 11, 2014.

18. Environmental Working Group, "Canaries in the Kitchen: Teflon Toxicosis," May 15, 2003, http://www.ewg.org/research/canaries-kitchen, accessed 6/21/17.

19. Environmental Working Group, "Canaries in the Kitchen: DuPont Has Known for 50 Years," May 15, 2003, http://www.ewg.org/research/canaries-kitchen/dupont-has-known-50-years, accessed 6/21/17.

20. R. Bressani, "Bean Grain Quality: A Review," *Archives of Latino American Nutrition* 39 (1989): 19–42.

21. S. K. Yadav and S. Sehgal, "Effect of Home Processing on Ascorbic Acid and Beta-Carotene Content of Spinach (*Spinacia oleracia*) and Amaranth (*Amaranthus tricolor*) Leaves," *Plant Foods in Human Nutrition* 47, no. 2 (1995): 125–131.

22. R. H. Liu, "Health Benefits of Fruit and Vegetables Are from Additive and Synergistic Combinations of Phytochemicals," *American Journal of Clinical Nutrition* 78, no. 3 (2003): 517S–520S.

23. "Lettuce Knives," *Cook's Illustrated*, July 2009.

INDEX

Fiber, types and nutritional benefits, 41
Fish and seafood
about: krill oil supplements, 55–56; omega-3 and -6 fats from, 44
Anchovy Dressing, 135
Broccoli Soup with Wild Hot Smoked Trout and Rosemary, 81
Fish Bone Broth, 91
Grilled Sardines with Chili, Oregano, and Lemon, 169
Keto Salad, 265
Scrambled Eggs with Smoked Trout and Herbs, 113–115
Whole Roasted Salmon with Lemon and Herbs, 194
Free radicals
carbs creating, 47
creation of, 5, 7, 35, 47
fasting benefits, 10
microwaves creating, 69
negative impact of, 5, 7
protection from, 58, 63
refined vegetable oil and, 35
as signaling molecules, 7
skipping dinner to reduce, 10
French fries, avoiding, 39–40
French Onion Soup, 92
Frittata with Loads of Veggies, 101
Fruit, eating organic, 19. See also Apple(s); Berries
Fudge, macadamia nut, 266

G

Garlic Confit, 254
GERD (Gastroesophageal reflux disease), 14
Ginger
Beef Broth with Turmeric, Coconut Cream, and Ginger, 78
Braised Ginger Chicken, 150
Coconut and Turmeric Kefir with Ginger and Cayenne, 202
Green Juice with Oil, 205
Indian Spice Dry Rub, 173
other recipes with, 85, 88–89, 124–125, 143, 159, 187, 193, 220
Turmeric, Lemon, and Ginger Juice with Oil, 214
Grains, avoiding, 38

Grass-Fed Beef Carpaccio with Celeriac Rémoulade, 166
Grass-Fed Steak with Chimichurri and Bone Marrow, 164–165
Gravy, roast beef and, 182–183
Green Juice with Oil, 205
Green Smoothie, 206
Grilled Sardines with Chili, Oregano, and Lemon, 169
Grilling guidelines and precautions, 65–67
Gypsy Salad, 139

H

Ham. See Pork
Hard-Boiled Eggs, 261
Herb Dressing, 242
Herb Oil, 247
Heterocyclic Amines (HCAs), 65–66, 67
Hydration. See Drinks

I

Iceberg Wedge Salad with Bacon and Egg, 140
Immune system, fasting benefitting, 11
Indian Spice Dry Rub, 173
Indian-Style Roast Chicken Drumsticks, 173
Inflammation, lowering, 5
Insulin
fasting benefits, 10–11
fat and, 28
lowering levels of, 6
monitoring blood sugar levels and, 23–24
protein intake and, 48
what it is and what it does, 3
Insulin resistance
beans, legumes and, 37
common to diseases, 3
cyclical nutritional ketosis reversing, 4–6
diabetes and, 21–22
diet and, 24
exercise and, 25
foods causing, 16
grains and, 38
leptin resistance and, 3, 4–6. See also Leptin resistance
microbe warding off, 17
milk, yogurt and, 37

processed fructose and, 34
ways to reduce, 17, 24, 25
weight loss and, 4–5, 31
Iodine supplements, 59–60

J

Jerusalem artichokes, braised lamb with, 153
Juniper berries, 126–127, 163

K

Kale
about: nutritional benefits, 45
Frittata with Loads of Veggies, 101
Green Juice with Oil, 205
Green Smoothie, 206
Kale and Pumpkin Tortilla, 105
Kale Caesar Salad, 144
Raw Beet Salad, 147
Kefir, coconut and turmeric with ginger and cayenne, 202
Keto Chocolate and Coconut Bites, 262
Keto Salad, 265
Ketogenic diet, cyclical. See also Nutrition, optimizing
benefits of, 4–6
fasting and, 10–12
low-carb, high-fat intake, 7–9
macronutrient ratios, 7–8
metabolism importance, 7–8
Mitochondrial Metabolic Therapy (MMT) and, 12
recipes in this book and, 72
reversing insulin/leptin resistance, 4–6
training body to recognize whole natural foods, 15
weight loss and, 4–5
when you eat, 9–10
Kimchi, 124–125
Knives, improving nutrient content, 71
Krauts. See Fermented foods
Krill oil supplements, 55–56

L

Lamb
about: AGEs and, 66
Braised Lamb with Jerusalem Artichokes, 153
Leaky gut syndrome, 15–16

ACKNOWLEDGMENTS

My deepest appreciation to Pete Evans for all his pioneering work in Australia to popularize this approach to eating and for helping to show how relatively easy it is to create healthy and delicious meals.

— DR. JOSEPH MERCOLA

I want to give a huge thanks to my loving family and to Dr. Mercola for all the support.

— PETE EVANS

ABOUT THE AUTHORS

Dr. Joseph Mercola

As a board-certified family physician for over three decades, Dr. Mercola treated many thousands of people at his wellness center where he focused on addressing the root cause of disease and encouraging patients to view food as medicine.

In 1997, he founded his website, Mercola.com, which has become the most visited natural-health website in the world and made him one of the leading teachers of health. Dr. Mercola's ultimate goal is to empower his millions of readers to take control of their health and to advocate for much-needed changes to our current health care system.

A best-selling author—most recently of the highly acclaimed *Fat for Fuel*—Dr. Mercola has appeared on CNN, Fox News, ABC News, *TODAY*, *Washington Unplugged*, and *The Dr. Oz Show*.

Website: www.mercola.com

Pete Evans

Pete Evans is an internationally renowned and household chef, restaurateur, author, and television presenter. His passion for food and a healthy lifestyle inspires individuals and families around the world.

Website: www.peteevans.com

HAY HOUSE TITLES OF RELATED INTEREST

YOU CAN HEAL YOUR LIFE, *the movie,* starring Louise Hay & Friends
(available as a 1-DVD program, an expanded 2-DVD set,
and an online streaming video)
Learn more at www.hayhouse.com/louise-movie

THE SHIFT, *the movie,* starring Dr. Wayne W. Dyer
(available as a 1-DVD program, an expanded 2-DVD set,
and an online streaming video)
Learn more at www.hayhouse.com/the-shift-movie

———

THE BONE BROTH SECRET: *A Culinary Adventure in
Health, Beauty, Longevity,* by Louise Hay and Heather Dane

CULTURED FOOD IN A JAR: *100+ Probiotic Recipes
to Inspire and Change Your Life,* by Donna Schwenk

THE REAL FOOD REVOLUTION: *Healthy Eating, Green Groceries,
and the Return of the American Family Farm,* by Congressman Tim Ryan

All of the above are available at your local bookstore,
or may be ordered by contacting Hay House (see next page).

———

We hope you enjoyed this Hay House book. If you'd like to receive our online catalog featuring additional information on Hay House books and products, or if you'd like to find out more about the Hay Foundation, please contact:

Hay House, Inc., P.O. Box 5100, Carlsbad, CA 92018-5100
(760) 431-7695 or (800) 654-5126
(760) 431-6948 (fax) or (800) 650-5115 (fax)
www.hayhouse.com® • www.hayfoundation.org

Published and distributed in Australia by:
Hay House Australia Pty. Ltd., 18/36 Ralph St., Alexandria NSW 2015
Phone: 612-9669-4299 • *Fax:* 612-9669-4144 • *www.hayhouse.com.au*

Published and distributed in the United Kingdom by:
Hay House UK, Ltd., Astley House, 33 Notting Hill Gate, London W11 3JQ
Phone: 44-20-3675-2450 • *Fax:* 44-20-3675-2451 • *www.hayhouse.co.uk*

Published and distributed in the Republic of South Africa by:
Hay House SA (Pty), Ltd., P.O. Box 990, Witkoppen 2068
info@hayhouse.co.za • *www.hayhouse.co.za*

Published in India by: *Hay House Publishers India,*
Muskaan Complex, Plot No. 3, B-2, Vasant Kunj, New Delhi 110 070
Phone: 91-11-4176-1620 • *Fax:* 91-11-4176-1630 • *www.hayhouse.co.in*

Distributed in Canada by:
Raincoast Books, 2440 Viking Way, Richmond, B.C. V6V 1N2
Phone: 1-800-663-5714 • *Fax:* 1-800-565-3770 • *www.raincoast.com*

<u>Access New Knowledge.</u>
<u>Anytime. Anywhere.</u>

Learn and evolve at your own pace with the world's leading experts.

www.hayhouseU.com

Free e-newsletters
from Hay House, the Ultimate
Resource for Inspiration

Be the first to know about Hay House's free downloads, special offers, giveaways, contests, and more!

 Get exclusive excerpts from our latest releases and videos from *Hay House Present Moments*.

 Our *Digital Products Newsletter* is the perfect way to stay up-to-date on our latest discounted eBooks, featured mobile apps, and Live Online and On Demand events.

 Learn with real benefits! *HayHouseU.com* is your source for the most innovative online courses from the world's leading personal growth experts. Be the first to know about new online courses and to receive exclusive discounts.

 Enjoy uplifting personal stories, how-to articles, and healing advice, along with videos and empowering quotes, within *Heal Your Life*.

 Have an inspirational story to tell and a passion for writing? Sharpen your writing skills with insider tips from *Your Writing Life*.

Sign Up Now!

Get inspired, educate yourself, get a complimentary gift, and share the wisdom!

Visit www.hayhouse.com/newsletters to sign up today!

 HAY HOUSE

 HAYHOUSE RADIO *radio for your soul®*

 HAYHOUSE online learning

Create a healthy, happy life with Hay House Online Learning

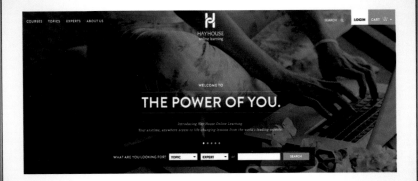

Visit www.hayhouseu.com/mercola to learn more about Dr. Mercola's MMT diet. We'll be featuring an in-depth, multi-lesson course that shows you how to bring everything you've learned in *Fat for Fuel* into your life.

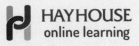